KITCHEN MAGIC

Keats Titles of Related Interest

Dr. Braly's Allergy and Nutrition Revolution
JAMES BRALY, M.D.

Allergy and Chinese Herbal Medicine
PI-KWANG TSUNG, PH.D.

Brain Allergies
WILLIAM H. PHILPOTT, M.D.
AND DWIGHT K. KALITA, PH.D.

Can A Gluten-Free Diet Help? How?
LLOYD ROSENVOLD, M.D.

Candida Albicans Yeast-Free Cookbook
PAT CONNOLLY

Do-It-Yourself Allergy Analysis Handbook
LOUISE HENDERSON, PH.D. AND KATE LUDEMAN, PH.D.

Gluten Intolerance
BEATRICE TRUM HUNTER

Good Food, Gluten-Free
HILDA CHERRY HILLS

Good Food, Milk-Free, Grain-Free
HILDA CHERRY HILLS

Good Food to Fight Migraine
HILDA CHERRY HILLS

If This Is Tuesday, It Must Be Chicken
NATALIE GOLOS AND FRANCES GOLOS GOLBITZ

Recognize and Manage Your Allergies
DORIS J. RAPP, M.D.

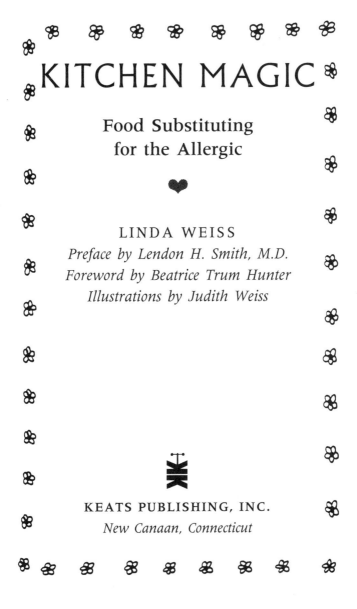

KITCHEN MAGIC

Food Substituting
for the Allergic

♥

LINDA WEISS

Preface by Lendon H. Smith, M.D.
Foreword by Beatrice Trum Hunter
Illustrations by Judith Weiss

KEATS PUBLISHING, INC.
New Canaan, Connecticut

Kitchen Magic is not intended as medical advice. Its intent is solely informational and educational. Please consult a health professional should a need for one be indicated.

KITCHEN MAGIC: Food Substituting for the Allergic

Library of Congress Cataloging-in-Publication Data

Weiss, Linda.
    Kitchen magic : food substituting for the allergic / Linda Weiss : illustrations by Judith Weiss.
        p.   cm.
    Includes index.
    ISBN 0-87983-636-9
    1. Ingredient substitutions (Cookery)   2. Food allergy—Diet therapy—Recipes.   I. Title.
    TX652.W385   1994
    641.5'63—dc20   94-25892
                                                              CIP

Printed in the United States of America

Book design by Joyce C. Weston

Published by Keats Publishing, Inc.
27 Pine Street (Box 876)
New Canaan, Connecticut 06840-0876

This book is lovingly dedicated to my eight-year-old
daughter Mia Dora, who waited, not always
so patiently, outside my office door and uttred these
immortal words each time I emerged,
"Can I bother you now?"

I expect I'll have many occasions to return
the favor when she becomes a teenager!

Acknowledgments

The encouragement I needed to write this book came from Janice Jones, R.N. in a unique way. She saw it completed while I still had it in my thoughts. Thank you, Jan.

The addition of some substitutions came to me from a very special lady, Kathleen Licari, who substitutes every day of her life. Thank you, Kathy.

The time I needed to complete this book was donated to me by husband, Milton, who still holds an I.O.U. Thank you, Milt.

To my good friend, Duane Karr, for lending me both of her hands, on a moment's notice. Thank you, Duane.

And to my mentor and very dear friend, Beatrice Trum Hunter, a very special thank you for sharing your eloquent thoughts and ideas with me during my moments of frustration and despair.

CONTENTS

PREFACE

It is a shame that we have to get sick so that we can find the path to health. Linda Weiss has been a victim of civilization and its "benefits." Her struggle to improve her immune system has netted us this fine book.

Many of us, maybe all of us, are victims of some food or chemical sensitivity. Strawberries will cause hives in some—usually the ones who love the red fruit. I get a nose bleed if I drink milk. Some get mean with a drive through traffic. Others will get depressed if they smell a certain perfume. When Ben Feingold found food sensitivities were the cause of much hyperactivity, we all felt it was but one or two percent, and the teachers noted that it was but one or two in every class. That was in 1950 that the teachers reported this low incidence. The decades and the pollution and the contamination of our food and atmosphere and water have increased apace. Now the teachers tell us that five to eight children in every class are so touched and, after Halloween and Easter, it shoots up to 90 percent of the class.

Even Scrooge thought some of his hallucinations were due to a bit of underdone potato. His cheerful demeanor on Christmas Day may have been the 12-hour fast he put himself on and then the good dinner he had at his nephew's.

Ecologically oriented health facilitators are gradually moving some of their patients from the psychiatrist's couches—those with fatigue or neurasthenia, those with psychosomatic stomachs, migraine, some of the arthritics, those with elevated blood pressure, some psychotics, and the best news of all, the hypochondriacs who knew there was something wrong. Because the examination and the laboratory reports show nothing really wrong, the doctor has no recourse but to label the patient as a psychiatric cripple. Maybe it's a Valium deficiency.

And now since we know that not everything can be blamed on your parents' poor nurturing skills, Linda gives us the practical way to recognize the symptoms and do something to get us out of the sickness mode. The disease that is due to a food or chemical sensitivity is a stress that depletes the immune system and thus makes the person more sensitive to weather changes, food additives, chlorine in the water and bad news.

Linda, with this great book, helps us all by making survival possible and better health attainable.

Lendon H. Smith, M.D.
author of *Feed Yourself Right,*
Feed Your Kids Right,
Dr. Lendon Smith's Low Stress Diet, and
Happiness Is a Healthy Life

FOREWORD

For individuals who need to make changes in food preparation in order to eliminate certain foods that are not tolerated, take heart. Help is on the way. Linda Weiss, who has gone through this experience, which can be overwhelming, has turned the obstacle into a challenge. In *Kitchen Magic* she demonstrates how favorite recipes can be adapted by substituting tolerated for non-tolerated ingredients. She provides many tempting and nutritious recipes, useful hints, and practical assistance with an up-to-date listing of sources for commercial products that might otherwise be difficult to locate.

Kitchen Magic will not only be helpful for those who must make adjustments in food preparation for reasons of health, but also offers an attractive assortment of recipes, from appetizers to desserts, that are wholesome and should have a wide general appeal. Weiss eliminates the confusion and bewilderment sometimes caused by the need for a sudden new approach to food preparation. She replaces the fear of being overwhelmed by her own special ingredient: her own easy-to-prepare approach.

—Beatrice Trum Hunter
author of *The Family Whole Grain Baking Book*

INTRODUCTION

❤ IN THE LIBRARY

I found hope in the library in a book called *An Alternative Approach to Allergies* by Theron Randolph M.D. and Ralph W. Moss Ph.D. I found out that I was not alone. In fact, in 1951, Dr. Randolph reported in his first book, *Human Ecology and Susceptibility to the Chemical Environment* that "seemingly harmless chemicals in use in our homes, offices, and work places every day in nontoxic doses were responsible for a wide variety of mental, emotional, and physical problems." He proposed alternative explanations and treatments for various diseases, both mental and physical. Dr. Randolph also reported that common foods were found to be the most frequent precipitating factors in environmental illness. Unfortunately, Dr. Randolph's book is relatively unknown to the general public and to much of the medical profession.

He wrote that a compromised immune system can mimic many illnesses and cause symptoms such as: sinus congestion, digestive disorders, joint and muscle weakness, spontaneous bruising, headaches, irritability, depression, dizziness, and fatigue . . . all of which I was experiencing. And if these symptoms are misdiagnosed, as is often the case, they can leave one vulnerable to many other diseases. Very often a person suffering from one or more of these systems is labeled "neurotic" by a well-meaning doctor who has not been trained to recognize multiple chemical sensitivity (MCS); or does not accept that physical symptoms can occur as a result of environmental exposures. And subsequently, without proper treatment, the victim may end up in a mental hospital, or at very best, feeling alone, depressed and left believing that he/she is mentally ill.

And today, further confusing the controversy over the existence of MCS, are Chronic Fatigue Syndrome (CFS) and Epstein-Barr Virus (EBV), two other recently acknowledged immune disorders with alarmingly similar symptomology. Very recently, these immune disorders, along with fibromyalgia (another disorder associated with CFS) and Acquired Immunodeficiency Syndrome (AIDS), are being grouped together and presented as Syndromes of Immune Disregulation (SID).

Dr. Randolph's book led me on a trip back in time, so I could trace the beginnings of the disease, and unravel the seemingly unrelated incidences of illness that were slowly diminishing my once radiant health. I hope the following account of my trip back to the future may help you to recognize your body's weaknesses, and that you may reclaim your health once you reach the point of no return.

❤ BACK TO THE FUTURE

"Eat your vegetables!" When I was a child, those three words ranked up there with "Do unto others as you would have others do unto you." I thought they were a part of grace, because they always followed "amen." That was in the 40's and 50's. Gardens were "in," and we grew a lot of our favorite vegetables in the vacant lot next door. Suburbs weren't overcrowded, so there were many vacant lots in the neighborhood. Unless you lived close to a factory, the air smelled fresh and clean. There weren't any toxic waste sites polluting our neighborhoods.

I used to hang around the kitchen a lot because it always smelled so good. Mothers cooked from scratch then. Microwave technology hadn't been tailor-made for home use yet, so we didn't eat nutritionally-empty dinners zapped in polystyrene foam throw-away containers. And there were no chemical fumes in the kitchen from heating plastic food wraps. "Landfill" was not yet a household word.

My dad was the official orange juicer at our house. Every morning we had fresh Florida orange juice, whether we wanted it or not. You might say he put the squeeze on us. Oranges were grown without the wide array of toxic chemicals, carcinogens, and mutagens used today.

We even had fresh milk delivered right to our doorstep in recyclable glass bottles every day, "from moo to you" as they used to say. Plastic bottles that leach chemicals into the milk were unheard of.

Fresh milk was the main ingredient in the ice cream we made. We used real eggs in the ice cream too, not the chemical egg replacer, diethyl glycol, as is commonly used in today's commercial brands. We had real vanilla on hand instead of piperonal, today's commercial alternative and a major ingredient in pesticides used to kill lice. We used real bananas instead of amyl acetate, which is a constituent in both paint and most commercial ice creams. Today, when you consume most commercial ice creams you're really eating a frozen chemical soup, unless you choose the chemical-free more natural ice creams now coming onto the market.

I remember being a typical, healthy youngster who loved playing baseball and volleyball. I was always on the go. I vividly remember my dad cornering me one day on the way out the door. In his most agitated voice, he blurted out, "We never see you anymore. You only come home to eat."

So what happened to my healthy body? Most would answer that question with "You're not as young as you used to be," or "Everybody gets something." But I'm not overweight. I'm still in my early fifties. I don't even *look* damaged. Not even in X-rays! The truth is that Multiple Chemical Sensitivity induced by modern technology is what happened to me. Television commercials primed me to believe that "you-name-it" Cola hit the spot and that "I deserved a break today." And I, like my peers, joined the fast-food lane in the 60's. I ate at restaurants often and became a pizza, hamburger, french fries, and hot fudge sundae junkie. I was unaware that I was ingesting an estimated 160 pounds per year of impairing additives in the form of preservatives, flavoring agents and dyes, along with my meals.

The adulteration of our food supply goes on and on, from irradiation of whole foods, antibiotics in livestock feed, lead in canned goods, preservatives in food packaging, and even threatened genetic changes in tomatoes, broccoli and cauliflower. Where will it end? As I am writing about how these so-called technological advances make our food unfit for human consumption, you can bet some chemist has just dreamed up yet another way to extend the shelf life of one more food product.

Then fast-food preparation hit the homefront.

Microwave mania overtook me and everyone else. We all became short order chefs. T.V. dinners and take-out hamburgers became the fast-food fare at home—a nutritional nightmare!

❤ THE CANCER PARADOX

As if this tampering with our foods wasn't enough, scientists were beginning to find new ways to dispose of chemicals that were developed for use in the jungles during World War II. Large stockpiles were left at the war's end, and a massive effort was launched, with the aid of the United States Department of Agriculture, to teach American farmers to use these chemicals for weed control.

One such compound is 2,4-Dichlorophenoxy acetic acid (2,4-D), a phenoxy herbicide. It is a component in the Vietnam War defoliant, Agent Orange, and is commonly used in about 1,500 lawn and garden products. Several studies link it to a type of lymph cancer. Many environmentalists and scientists attribute 2,4-D to causing birth defects, liver cancer and neurological damage.

And other compounds, such as organochlorines, are regularly used in lawns and gardens. Two such organochlorines that are known animal carcinogens are PCB and DDT, which have been banned for use in the U.S. Yet even today, third world countries use DDT in their growing fields, then ship their product to the United States. So we continue to ingest banned DDT, when we consume the many imported fruits and vegetables purchased in our grocery stores.

DDT and PCB's have been found in human fat tissue, but until recently their association with human cancer occurrence has only been marginally studied. However, in a study reported in *The Journal of the National Cancer Institute* (Vol. 85, No. 8) states, "Our data suggest that organochlorine residues and, in particular, DDE, a metabolite of DDT, are strongly associated with breast cancer risk."

Many other pesticide residues are found in U.S.-grown produce. In a recent analysis of a National Academy of Sciences report, indications are that "millions of children in the U.S. receive up to 35% of their entire lifetime dose of some carcinogenic pesticides by age 5."

Since pesticides reside in fat cells, one might further speculate that animals raised on sprayed feed accumulate pesticides in their fat tissues. Then, when we ingest meat and milk products, especially fatty cheese and whole milk made from those animals, we may be receiving another dose of chemicals which are known to promote cancer. Might the missing link in the fat/cancer relationship be due to a weakened immune system caused by eating and breathing so many of these man-made chemicals?

❤ WHAT DO WE DO NOW?

For the past several years, doctors have been advising us to eat certain kinds of vegetables and to cut down on fat consumption as a means of obtaining optimum health, without realizing that our foods have been grown in over-chemicalized, minerally-depleted soil. And depleted soil produces nutritionally empty food. Might this be another missing link?

Food researchers know food value losses are inevitable after harvest. It has been reported that 10 percent of a food's nutritional value will be lost when the food is first removed from the growing field. Another 10 percent will be lost during shipping, and another 10 percent will be lost in storage and display at the retail level. Another 10 percent will be lost in home storage, and still another 10 percent or more, will be lost in cooking and processing at home . . . and the picture gets bleaker.

The next step in food processing might be heating, canning, freezing, pickling, irradiating, or one of many others. During these various food processing methods, much of a food's original value is diminished. Where does all this leave us? Eating food that has been robbed of many nutrients. So if you're like most Americans, relying on frozen orange juice shipped in from Brazil (where DDT is still legal) to meet your Recommended Dietary Allowance (RDA) of vitamin C, you've been misled.

Just to refresh your memory, the scenario thus far: chemical applications on foods; poor nutritional content of soil; many types of food processing; and in some instances chemically contaminated air. They all play havoc with our health.

There is yet another important factor missing. We aren't healthy one day and sick the next. Becoming ill is a gradual process, and misdiagnosed and misunderstood minor ailments may become major diseases. And that is exactly what happened to me, a gradual breakdown of my immune system, misdiagnosed for perhaps as long as five years, led to Multiple Chemical Sensitivity. MCS is one of the most misdiagnosed and least understood diseases of the 20th century, the disease that will take us all "back to the future."

❤ MY EARLY SYMPTOMS OF IMMUNE SYSTEM BREAKDOWN

The first misdiagnosed sign of MCS for me was a spastic colon, the name given to most unremarkable intestinal ailments. This went on for several years and my internist prescribed a muscle relaxant and antacids as needed, since the head-to-toe physical examination and X-rays revealed no obvious medical problem. "It's just a case of nervous tension," he assured me. I reluctantly acquiesced.

The next symptom appeared while in my dentist's office. I nearly passed out after an injection of novocaine. I went limp and the dentist used smelling salts to revive me. He then suggested that I must have been apprehensive about "the needle." I was doubtful, but accepted his scenario of the incident.

Over the next several years, I began suffering from a plethora of minor ailments, from bouts of sinus congestion to heart palpitations. I noticed an occasional metallic taste in my mouth. Abdominal symptoms remained a constant companion, and I had begun to take for granted the regimen of "nerve pills" and antacids. Then, when frequent one-sided headaches became the norm at work, I accepted the doctor's diagnosis of nervous tension and decided to take a vacation.

While on my vacation, my weakened immune system finally gave out and exhaust fumes, perfumes, and cigarette smoke suddenly became intolerable. My husband had to carry me out of a shopping mall when I suddenly became too weak to walk. I finally knew what it was like to "shop till you drop." When I collapsed while walking across a golf course, I knew something terrible was happening to me. Our vacation came to an abrupt halt and the next three months were spent in a local library researching my symptomology. It was there that I began to find some answers.

When I left the library with Dr. Randolph's book under my arm, I knew what I had to do: find a doctor who practices environmental medicine. This new breed of doctor was a rarity in 1981, but by calling the American Academy of Environmental Medicine in Denver, Colorado, I located Dr. Paula Davey, a gastroenterologist and a clinical ecologist practicing in Ann Arbor, Michigan, about an hour from my home.

During the three month time lapse between "knowing" I had a misdiagnosed physical problem and in receiving treatment, I became an environmental cripple. My stomach problems were exacerbated, and the more I ate, the weaker I became.

I was truly frightened the day of my first grueling four hour appointment with Dr. Davey. But, two weeks later, after a complete environmental workup, including a childhood illness history, numerous blood tests, and "provocative" food and chemical testing, I at last received a diagnosis other than "nerves." "You have multiple chemical sensitivities," the doctor explained. "It means that your body's defense mechanisms are not able to protect you against the unavoidable chemicals in your food, water, and air. The tests also indicate that you have subsequently developed allergies to 85 foods. Maldigestion which leads to malabsorption of food, is brought on by chemical exposure, and is thought to be one of the major causes of multiple chemical sensitivity. We can try to rebuild your immune system, but it will take a serious commitment on your part. It took a long time to reach this point, and it will take a long time to reverse the damage, but it can be done!"

I accepted "the challenge" on the spot. It would require me to follow a rotation diet (a diet which prevents one from eating from the same food families oftener than once every 5 to 7 days); eat only organic foods; rely heavily on vitamin and mineral supplementation; and provide a "safe haven"—a place somewhere in the home that is totally free of chemicals. I was willing to do *anything* this doctor advised me to do. She believed in me. She offered me a future. I found myself throwing my arms around her for having the courage to add these innovative techniques to her medical practice and for her resolve to help others like myself, who were being written off as hypochondriacs. This was the beginning of my long, difficult road "back to the future."

Imagine thanking a person who has just told you to change your entire lifestyle by eating only organic, unprocessed food, wearing only untreated cotton or silk clothing, drinking filtered water, removing carpeting, upholstered furniture, and any synthetic bedding from your home. And if possible, have your gas furnace converted to electric! It meant stripping my home of most modern conveniences and a lifetime of accumulations! I did it all, and I've never regretted any of it. Although I shed some tears while packing up my entire wardrobe of synthetics and placing everything made out of plastic or vinyl in storage. I was convinced that I would be well enough to use them again in the future. And since this was only a temporary measure, one that was necessary to regain my health, I considered it a "treatment," and carried on like a trouper.

I made astounding physical improvements in my "safe house." Chronic abdominal symptoms subsided, due to my dietary changes. My sinus ailments cleared up. Even the throaty "ahems" that had promptly followed all my meals disappeared. I had expected to have sinus problems my entire life! I had been under the impression that sinus problems were due to weather conditions. How silly of me.

With my food allergens weeded out, and while living in a chemical-free indoor environment, my energy level bounced back quickly. So I began walking for exercise. But a rude awakening was yet to come.

It seems that during the healing crisis, the less toxic you become the more sensitive you temporarily become to offending substances. One day while out walking by many freshly pesticided lawns, I became ill. I became disoriented repeatedly during my walks and began having severe heart palpitations that on one occasion required a rescue squad to revive me. When passing freshly asphalted roads I experienced the same symptoms. After these exposures, I became so sensitive I could no longer tolerate prescribed nutrients. To say I became despondent is putting it mildly. My life was becoming more like a never-ending nightmare.

There would be many more visits to Dr. Davey with many more questions, all the time wondering if I would ever heal. I still thank God for her patience, her understanding, and her conviction that I would keep improving, despite these small setbacks that felt like major hurdles to me. Each time she gave me new found strength. And each time my husband, an organic gardener, backed her up, held me up, and kept me "growing."

During the ceaseless process of removing "chemical excitants" from my life, the most difficult of all to give up was makeup, hairspray, and other beauty products. Until this time my losses were all material. They were replaceable objects that once out of sight, became out of mind. But this was more difficult. To say "I had to meet the real me on this long road back to health" would be a fair statement. But I soon realized that there is life after makeup.

Following my terrifying walking experiences and several other defeats wreaked by modern technology, I became pretty much the recluse that the illness dictated. But, being the devout social animal that I am, I sneaked out occasionally when someone could accompany me in case of trouble. Yet, it would be a very long time before I ventured out completely on my own.

Sometime during the next year, I realized that I had slowly, out of necessity, become an expert at finding alternative ways of healthy living and cooking. I began to risk taking assisted outings more often, and for longer periods of time. My immune system was beginning to come to my defense. I even managed to conjure up gourmet meals using ingredients that I had only recently learned to pronounce.

Rapidly, word spread amongst an ever-growing community of chemically sensitive persons, that I could help find hard to locate products and foods that were free of toxic chemicals. It was then, as I began to help others find alternative products, that I decided to turn this illness and all its limitations into an ally. I decided to catalog all the foodstuffs, alternative healthcare, clothing, household and cleaning products that made living easier for me. And with Dr. Davey's assistance, my first book, a self-help resource guide, "How To Live With The New 20th Century Illness," was born. This was my debut as a writer.

Somewhere between the search for alternative healthcare products and the publishing of my first book, having a made-up face lost its importance. I had lost my severe case of "vanityitis," and I knew that the nightmare, although by no means over, would have a happy ending. Perhaps this was God's way of getting my attention and giving me something much more important to do. And, as if "from my thoughts to God's ears" that realization led to an opportunity to write an alternative healthcare column, called "Healthwatch," in a local newspaper.

My advice column caught the eyes of readers across the country; then when I received letters from Canada and England, I knew that people all over the world were experiencing health problems from chemical exposures of one kind or another. This gave me the incentive to keep writing. I knew I was in the right place at the right time.

During this time, as my food allergies continued to improve along with my overall health, I began experimenting with more alternative methods of food preparation. I had always been comfortable in the kitchen, and since I still remained confined to my house a lot, this seemed to be an opportune time to become a creative cook again. Besides, I missed eating quiche, lasagna, chopped liver, and chocolate mousse. Being allergic to beef, wheat, and chocolate wasn't going to stop me now, not after all I'd been through!

Kitchen Magic is the result of my life-threatening experiences and of going "back to the future" in order to survive the present artificial world we live in. For those of you who are already dealing with chemical and food sensitivities and for those of you who hope to avoid them, you will find that it's easier than you think, once you have the tools to work with.

HOW TO USE THIS GUIDE

Do you believe in magic? I do—the magic of substitution. With this guide, you will be able to take your favorite recipes, replace the offending ingredients, and *voilà*—even a member of the family relegated to a special diet will be able to enjoy the same dinner! No more cooking separate dishes with someone feeling left out. Not only will the taste be fantastic, but cooking more chemically-free and using whole grains, natural sweeteners and organic produce when available, will certainly promote a healthier family.

In some areas I have given you alternatives that may be used but are definitely less desirable for health reasons. I have included them, however, because someone may have a severe allergy problem, and that may be the only alternative for them.

Just as a magician has props to captivate his audience so that they continually have pleasing objects and colors to look at, so must a cook. Eye appeal is so very important, as it can make the diner feel he is eating at the most elegant restaurant. A simple slice of orange or apple, a radish flower, or even a few slices of cucumber placed strategically on a plate (keeping an eye out for color combination) can transform a simple omelet into a delightful entrée.

If you use serving dishes at the table, try using several different shapes and sizes, always choosing a dish to fit the food. A half-empty serving dish makes one wonder if the cat got there first!

Once you have your diners' eye appeal, the rest will be easy. Just turn the pages and learn how your labor of love will give someone you love a joyous appetite again! So don't be afraid to be a kitchen magician and start substituting right now.

I have included many of my favorite recipes to help you get started. As soon as you get the hang of it, you will be creating your own unique palate pleasers, and through the magic of substitution you too will become a kitchen magician.

SECTION ONE

GETTING STARTED

❤ COOKING WITHOUT CHEMICALS

If you're green inside, you're clean inside! So, eat as many raw fruits and vegetables as possible. Raw food is still living food. It is not dead, it has just stopped growing. Avoid highly processed foods because the food value has been diminished.

Consume foods labeled "organic" whenever possible since these products have been grown without the use of chemical sprays and fertilizers. Be skeptical of foods labeled "natural—no chemicals or preservatives added." This may merely mean that nothing has been added after the food was picked. Chances are that chemicals were used while the food was still growing in the field. Any food that has been aged in any way (pickled, smoked, fermented or dried) has mold in it or on it. Many spices are also heavily contaminated with pesticides. Some are irradiated to kill insects and bacteria. Some of these condiments are also actually irritating to the stomach lining, weaken the system, and contaminate the blood. For these reasons, it is best to grow your own herbs like basil, thyme, rosemary, and parsley.

It is estimated that 850 million pounds of pesticides and herbicides, not to mention another 22.3 billion pounds of fertilizers, are used on food crops. And with consumption of fresh fruits and vegetables increasing, it is possible that we are being poisoned at the dinner table. The concern is with the possible side effects that stem from a lifetime of eating chemically treated produce.

In addition to these chemicals, some produce undergoes further cosmetic treatment. Beeswax and paraffin are relatively non-toxic, but vinyl chloride polymer, classed among human carcinogens, can also be used to embalm fruits and vegetables. The waxes are used to reduce water loss and to enhance the appearance of the produce. Often, the waxes have several potentially dangerous fungicides added to them, a discomforting thought since not all of the waxes can be completely washed off.

Many of the chemicals used in growing produce are systemic and cannot be removed by washing. But some of the surface residues on produce can be removed by using the following simple methods:

Wash produce in a solution of one-fourth cup of three percent food grade hydrogen peroxide (H_2O_2) to a sink full of cold water. Soak light vegetables similar to lettuce and other greens 20 minutes; thicker skinned vegetables, like cucumbers 30 minutes. Rinse and dry thoroughly and refrigerate.

Although much nutritional value will be lost, peeling fruits and vegetables is another alternative.

Buy domestically grown produce and produce in season, preferably grown close to home, to eliminate extra chemical treatments. And beware of flawless produce; it is apt to be the most contaminated.

❤ LESS TOXIC COOKWARE AND FOOD STORAGE

Use glass, porcelain or stainless steel cookware. Non-stick coatings contain fluorocarbons that can leach out into your food. Corning cookware can be special ordered without the non-stick coating. (See Product Guide page 202.) Steaming is the least allergenic way to cook. So, steam foods instead of boiling, whenever possible. Lightly stir-frying is also a good alternative. Remember, the less cooking the more nutrition retained.

Be especially careful when using Silverstone and Teflon not to let them boil dry. Toxic fumes may be released from them at temperatures above 400°. After 20 minutes this release is enough to make a person ill. Birds and other pets are particularly susceptible.

Microwave cooking? The jury is still out on this. If used, purchase a microwave oven with leaded walls so the microwaves cannot escape.

Store foodstuffs in unbleached paper or glass containers instead of plastic bags. Cellophane is okay—it is made from cellulose which is a plant derivative. But don't buy foods embalmed in heat-sealed plastic packages. During processing the heat causes the plastic molecules to become permanently impregnated into the contents. When you have a choice, purchase liquids in glass containers rather than plastic or waxed cardboard to prevent toxins from leaching into the contents. Food purchased in a tied, plastic package can be transferred to a glass, ceramic or stainless steel container. After letting the contents air out for three days, it will be ready to use.

Most commercial wax paper, napkins, paper towels, coffee filters, and baking cups are bleached. Chlorine-based chemicals like dioxin, considered to be one of the most deadly chemicals known to science, are commonly used in this process. These chemicals are then dumped into our lakes and streams.

So purchase 100 percent unbleached, undyed paper products for use in the kitchen whenever possible. See Product Guide, page 202.

By choosing to use these unbleached paper products, you are being kind to the environment and preventing your food from coming in contact with chemicals remaining on the food wrap. This is especially important when reheating or baking foods in paper products.

❤ FOOD IRRADIATION

Food irradiation is a process which kills insects and microorganisms on foods by zapping the foods with streams of gamma radiation from recycled radioactive cobalt-60 and cesium-137. Although the foods do not become radioactive, some of their cells undergo chemical changes.

The chemical changes produce new chemical substances called Radiolytic Products (RP's) and substances known as Unique Radiolytic Products (URP's)—substances that would not be in the food had it not been irradiated. Examples of these substances are formaldehyde, benzene, and peroxide. The long-term biological effects of the URP's are unknown and inadequately investigated.

Who advocates food irradiation? Early on, the most aggressive irradiation advocates were the U.S. Army and the Atomic Energy Commission (AEC), later reorganized as the Nuclear Regulatory Commission. In the early 1960's the intention was to preserve foods permanently for shipping to the front-line troops. When various tests revealed extensive damage to laboratory animals fed irradiated food (e.g. abnormal eyes, hemorrhages, and hearts with enlarged left ventricles) experimenters began to use lower doses of radiation and lowered their sights to longer shelf-life, instead of permanent preservation.

Some say that the intention now is to reduce substantially the disposal cost of nuclear plant wastes. This merely would shift the problem of waste disposal from the nuclear power plants to the food irradiation facilities.

Irradiation has been in use for some time for spices at the wholesale level, although irradiation of wheat and potatoes was approved long ago, for export only. More recently, poultry, pork, onions, and garlic were added to the list of approved foods for radiation treatment.

In 1986, the FDA legalized irradiation of certain fresh fruits and vegetables and tripled the dose previously allowed on spices.

Is irradiated food safe to eat? Some studies suggest that it is, while other studies suggest that irradiated foods are linked to kidney and liver disease, mutations, cancer, and other health problems.

Beatrice Trum Hunter, food editor of *Consumer's Research* magazine, states that, "Although irradiated chicken resists salmonella, there are radiation resistant bacteria. The bacteria that causes botulism resists radiation, and the elimination of competing bacteria could cause what has been termed 'microbial havoc'."

The dosages of irradiation allowed on fresh fruits and vegetables are up to a kiloGray, equivalent to 30 million chest x-rays, and the allowable dosage on herbs and spices is up to 30 kiloGrays.

Why aren't retail foods labeled as such? Only irradiated foods shipped in bulk to a processor for further processing must bear a label that states: "Treated with ionizing radiation—do not irradiate again." Whole food items that are sold at the retail level to consumers are required to be labeled "treated with radiation." To date, there is an extremely limited number of treated foods reaching the American marketplace. The FDA does not have enough inspectors to police the radiation industry. The agency is concerned that food labeled "treated with radiation" would adversely affect consumer acceptance.

So how do you avoid buying irradiated foods? The only way to determine if the food you purchase has been irradiated, is to buy food labeled "not irradiated." Usually, such food is organically grown as well. Be sure to tell your grocer that you would not purchase irradiated food. Grass roots efforts *do* make a difference.

❤ A WORD ABOUT COMMERCIAL MEAT

Today an estimated 50 percent of the antibiotics manufactured in the United States are fed to, injected into or applied to livestock. Even after slaughter, the chemical treatments may continue. At the supermarket, steaks, chops and roasts are sometimes dipped into antibiotic solutions or chemical preservatives to increase shelf life.

If you're allergic to antibiotics you may have severe reactions to the residues of these drugs in the animal products you consume. There are currently 20,000 to 30,000 animal drugs in use today, some of which are hormones and pesticides. Some of them present a potential cancer risk to humans.

In the late 1980s, a discovery by the Atlanta Center for Disease Control added fuel to an old controversy over the practice of raising animals on drug-enriched feed. Researchers, headed by epidemiologist Scott Holmberg, proved that the overuse of antibiotics spawned new kinds of bacteria in cattle who then developed a resistance to these so-called "wonder drugs." Holmberg and his colleagues also proved that there was a link between these new forms of bacteria in cattle and antibiotic-resistant bacteria subsequently found in humans. The most common of these is a form of salmonella found in beef, milk, and eggs that does not respond to normal treatment with antibiotics. This strain of bacteria causes nearly 36,000 cases of diarrhea annually in the United States.

To avoid this risk to your health, purchase organic meat, eggs and poultry that are grown without the use of these drugs. It is also important to follow a few simple sanitary procedures when handling raw meat, especially chicken and eggs.

Wash your hands before and after handling raw meat or poultry. Cook the meat thoroughly; high temperatures kill the bacteria. Use soap and water to clean all surfaces and utensils that have come in contact with the raw meat or poultry during food preparation. Wash eggshells with soap and water before cracking.

❤ BUTTER AND OILS

As an important health measure, avoid hydroge-nated (hardened) or partially hydrogenerated fats and oils such as margarine, shortenings, and fac-tory-produced foods to which these modified oils and fats have been added. They are difficult to digest, and interfere with normal cell metabolism. Research has shown that this interference with normal cell function may be a contributing factor to heart disease and cancer. It is advisable to reduce your intake of hydrogenated oils and fats whenever possible.

What about polyunsaturated fats? Too much

polyunsaturated fat in your diet may also increase your cancer risk, some experts say. So moderation is the key, until the fat facts are all in. However, the experts do agree that not more than 30 percent of our daily calories should be from fats; and only 10 percent of that should be from saturated fats. Fats are essential in your body for hormone production, protein metabolism, and to increase the integrity of cell membranes (our first defense against bacterial and viral infection). Liquid vegetable oils are your best option.

Unrefined, cold-pressed oils, which can be purchased at health food stores, can be used successfully for all of your baking and cooking needs. Cold-pressed oils are extracted by mechanical pressing, without the use of chemicals. Because these oils have not been exposed to high temperatures they are full of nutrients, unlike the chemically refined cooking oils you will find at most grocery stores. The vegetable oils available at most grocery stores have been extracted using petroleum solvents, with the addition of preservatives, anti-foaming agents, and many other additives. They are refined by heat, which devitalizes fat and causes oxidation, and thus rancidity.

Since not all vegetable oils contain the same amounts of saturated, polyunsaturated, and monounsaturated fatty acids, it would be prudent to consume those that have the highest concentration of monounsaturated fats. They are the ones that have been touted as the "good guys." Beware of partially hydrogenated oils often found in processed food. They contain trans fatty acids which can raise cholesterol levels.

Monounsaturated fats, unlike polyunsaturated and saturated fats, help reduce the artery-clogging kind of cholesterol. Some of the recommended monounsaturated vegetable oils are sesame, peanut, high-oleic safflower, high-oleic sunflower, canola, and olive oil. Of these, olive oil is a favorite of mine, due to its unique flavor and aroma. I use only organic, extra-virgin olive oil which is also cold-pressed. Studies show that the Mediterraneans, who have been indulging in large quantities of olive oil for many generations, have a lower cancer and heart attack risk than Americans do. Olive oil also has a greater resistance to oxidation.

Canola oil is one of the latest additions to the monounsaturated class of vegetable oils. It is a rapeseed oil product of Canada that has had most of the erucic acid removed. It contains only a very small percentage of erucic acid, but this acid has been found to be toxic. For this reason, and because most canola oil is highly refined, I have reservations about using it.

All oils should be refrigerated after opening to reduce the risk of light-induced rancidity. At the risk of repeating myself, an extra word of caution when purchasing cooking oils—go organic. If the final verdict comes in and pesticides are a big part of the fat/cancer connection, then you'll be thankful you made the change.

❤ FAKE FAT—COMMERCIAL SUBSTITUTES I DON'T RECOMMEND

I feel it's important to mention the most recent alternative fat temptations that are bound to add confusion to an already dizzying fat story. *Olestra* and *Simplesse* are being called worry-free fake fats and are being touted as desirable fat substitutes. According to the Monsanto Company, manufacturers of Simplesse, it can be used in place of oil-based products, such as margarine and salad dressing, and can be used in place of fat in all dairy products. It is made from natural protein found in egg whites or milk. If on a protein restricted diet, or, if allergic to milk or eggs, you may want to avoid Simplesse.

Proctor and Gamble's phony fat, Olestra, a sucrose-polyester, is made by altering the natural makeup of fat. This change allows the fat to pass through your body without being absorbed, rendering it fat-free. P&G says Olestra can be substituted for up to 35 percent of the fat in shortenings and cooking oils, and can replace up to 75 percent of the fat used for commercial deep fat frying.

Trailblazer, another fake fat, made from egg and milk protein, is manufactured by Kraft General Foods.

But are these new technologies safe? P&G's studies have shown that Olestra causes cancer, liver damage, and other disorders in animals, reports the Center for Science in the Public Interest, a non-profit consumer group based in Washington D.C. They further point to other studies which indicate that fat-soluble vitamins will be removed with Olestra as it leaves the body.

You can avoid consuming these fake fats by reading labels carefully. For example, Simple Pleasures, a substitute ice cream, contains Simplesse.

FOOD GLOSSARY

All of these products are available through health food stores and are sometimes carried in well-stocked supermarkets or Oriental food markets. Refer to page 196 for a complete list of products.

Acerola Cherry Powder: A powder made from dried and ground berries of the acerola plant. This powder is a very rich natural source of vitamin C. One-half teaspoon contains 85 mg of C. Used as a vitamin supplement or as a tea substitute.

Agar-Agar: A sea vegetable used to jell liquid. It is available in cakes and sticks and is as simple to use as gelatin. High in calcium and magnesium, low in fat and calories.

Amaranth Flour: Amaranth was known as the "wonder grain" by the Aztecs. It is rich in calcium, iron, and phosphorus, and contains lysine, one of the eight essential amino acids. It contains little fat and combines well with other flours when used in baking. Amaranth seeds may be added when baking breads. Amaranth flakes are becoming a popular cereal.

Arrowroot Flour (Starch): A tropical plant whose root is finely ground and used as a thickening agent for making gravies, puddings and sauces. Do not use arrowroot in a recipe that has to be rewarmed as it loses its thickening capacity.

Artichoke Flour (Starch): Made from grinding dried Jerusalem artichokes. May be used in making a milk substitute. Sometimes found in pasta.

Barley Malt: Fermented barley made by soaking and sprouting the barley. The end result is malt. Another portion of barley is then added and cooked until the starch is converted to sugar. Available as syrup or powder, and used as a sweetener in baking.

Brewer's Yeast: Brewer's yeast is a nutritional yeast grown on molasses. It contains all of the essential amino acids, B vitamins and minerals. It can be purchased in flake or powder form.

Brown Rice Syrup Powder: A crystallized form of brown rice syrup and natural enzymes that has been ground to a very fine powder. Imparts a very light sweet taste that can be used as a sugar substitute.

Buckwheat Groats: Buckwheat is often incorrectly thought to be a member of the grass family, but it is actually a herbaceous plant from an entirely different botanical family. The fruits are commonly called buckwheat groats and may be ground into a flour or cooked and used as a cereal or a porridge, which is called kasha.

Carob Powder: Ground from the pod-like fruit of the carob tree. Because it is high in calcium and phosphorus, low in fat, and caffeine free, it has become very desirable in baking as a chocolate substitute. It is also available as carob chips, chunks and syrup. Carob powder is available in pure form. However, carob chips usually contain sweeteners and fats. Carob syrup has many additives.

Cream of Tartar: A product of the grape family and the acid ingredient necessary for the release of carbon dioxide gas from baking soda. It is used in making your own baking powder.

Date Sugar: Ground, dried dates, a little less sweet than white sugar. It has many varied uses.

Essene Bread: Or Bible bread, as it is sometimes called. Made from sprouted grain which is ground to a doughy consistency, then shaped into loaves, and baked at low temperatures until crusty on the outside with a moist, chewy inside. Seeds, nuts and fruits are sometimes added. Nutritionally, Essene bread is an abundant source of vitamins, minerals, fiber, protein and natural sugars. The many enzymes present in the sprouts make the nutrients easy to digest.

Flaxseeds: Seeds of the flax plant. They are high in healthful unsaturated fatty acids, minerals and protein. Used as an egg substitute in baking.

Fruitsource Sweetener: An unrefined sweetener available in liquid and granular forms made from fruit juice (grapes) and complex carbohydrates (whole rice). Used in place of sugar or as a substitute for molasses and honey.

Garbanzo Flour: Finely ground garbanzo beans used in baking as a flour and as an egg substitute.

Ghee: Clarified butter. Used for centuries in India and in the Middle East. Does not bubble or smoke when heated and contains no additives, yet does not turn rancid. Made from cow's milk, but is virtually lactose-free. Use in place of regular butter for cooking.

Goat's Milk: May be purchased raw or pasteurized and in liquid or dry form. Some people tolerate the lactalbumin, a protein in goat's milk because it differs from the lactalbumin in cow's milk.

Kamut Flour: An ancient, highly nutritious wheat flour that contains more protein, minerals, and amino acids than common wheat. Kamut also contains a different type of gluten which is easier for the body to utilize. Some persons allergic to wheat can tolerate kamut. Also available as a puffed cereal.

Kefir: A fermented milk made with bacterial cultures similar to that of yogurt, used as a drink and in desserts. Produces less lactose than similar dairy products.

Kefir Cheese: Made from kefir milk that has had the water removed. Used as a sour cream alternative and as a spread.

Kelp Powder: A dark green seaweed that is high in iodine and other minerals. Used as a tenderizer when cooking beans and as a table salt substitute although it is not low in sodium.

Kuzu Root Starch: An excellent thickener in cooking that is easily prepared. Often mixed with potato starch, so if you have a potato allergy, make sure the package is labeled 100% Kuzu.

Lecithin, Liquid: Lecithin oil is derived from soybeans. It acts as an emulsifier, breaking down fat. It can be used as a lubricant for pans in baking, and also acts as a preservative. May also be purchased in granular form.

Liquid Aminos: A liquid form of vegetable protein from soybeans. Loaded with vitamins and minerals. Used to replace tamari and soy sauce. Also used to flavor soups, tofu, and vegetables.

Maple Syrup Granules: A dry form of pure maple syrup which has only the water removed from it, leaving it in a convenient dry form to use as granulated sugar.

Matzoh: A yeast-free, milk-free, whole wheat or unbleached wheat flour cracker used as a baking substitute in pie crusts, and as a breading.

Matzoh Meal: A meal made by pulverizing unbleached matzoh. May be used as a bran substitute or as a breading.

Milk, Powdered: Made by removing at least 95% of the water from either whole or skimmed milk. Spray-dried powdered milk remains the most nutritious powdered milk due to its low-heat processing. It is available in goat's milk, soy, yogurt or buttermilk, skim or whole, instant or non-instant. Has as many varied uses as regular milk.

Millet: A grain which can be purchased whole, cracked or ground as a flour. It is a more complete protein than any other grain, is particularly high in minerals, and is easy to digest. As a grain it is used in cereals, puddings, and as a rice substitute. As a flour, it is used in baking.

Miso: Made by crushing boiled soybeans, and adding barley, rice or wheat. Misos are complete proteins and rich in calcium, phosphorus, and B vitamins. Their beneficial digestive enzymes are similar to those found in yogurt and other fermented foods. Add at end of cooking since boiling destroys the enzymes. Used in soups as a flavoring, or mixed with nut butters as a spread for toast. Also a good salt substitute, though still high in sodium.

Molasses: Most molasses is a by-product of white sugar manufacturing. Blackstrap molasses, a thick, dark syrup produced during the refinement of sugar contains a valuable amount of minerals. Unfortunately, it also contains a high concentration of pesticides and chemical residues from the refining process. Used as a sweetener in baking.

Mung Bean Threads: Thin spaghetti-like noodles made of mung bean starch and commonly used in Oriental cooking.

Oat Bran: The ground husk layers of oats that contain most of the nutrients and fiber. Used as a cereal or a substitute for wheat bran.

Potato Flour (Starch): Prepared from dehydrated potatoes. It is especially suited for baking and as a thickening agent in pies and fruit sauces.

Pumpkin Seeds: The highly nutritious seed of the pumpkin. May be ground and used like peanut butter.

Quinoa: An ancient wheat-free and gluten-free grain known by the Incas as "The Mother

Grain." Usually combined with corn flour when made into pasta. Also available as a cereal.

Rice Bran: The ground husk layers of rice that contain most of the nutrients and fiber. Used as a wheat bran substitute.

Rice Cakes: A thick cracker, approximately 1/2", made from whole grain brown rice and, usually, salt. Can also be purchased with the addition of buckwheat, sesame seeds or millet. They are especially tasty spread with nut butters and/or preserves.

Rice Noodles: Thin spaghetti-like noodles made of rice starch; commonly used in Oriental cooking.

Rice Vinegar: Fermented brown or white rice and water. If brown rice is used, the vinegar will be amber colored instead of clear. Rice vinegar is low in acid and therefore desirable.

Sea Salt: Seawater that has been vacuum dried. It contains calcium chloride as well as other sea minerals. Used as a table salt substitute, although it is still high in sodium.

Slippery Elm Powder: Made from the bark of the Slippery Elm tree. It is used as an egg replacer.

Spelt Flour: Although a member of the wheat family, this European grain can often be tolerated by wheat sensitive individuals. It is similar to hard wheat and is used in bread baking. Also available as a cereal.

Sorghum Molasses: The result of pressing, evaporating, and then slow cooking the juice from the green stalks of sorghum cane. Used as a sweetener in baking.

Soy Flour: Made from ground soybeans, which contain the most protein of any bean. Soy flour has no gluten so it cannot be used alone to make bread, but it makes a great high-protein addition to other flours in baking. It is also used as an egg yolk substitute, and in making a milk substitute.

Soy Milk: The liquid pressed from ground, cooked soy beans, high in vegetable protein. Usually contains an added sweetener. Used for drinking and in cooking.

Soy Yogurt: Made from soy milk with the addition of a bacterial culture. It is used as an alternative to cow's or goat's milk yogurt for dietary purposes.

Sucanat: 100 percent evaporated organic sugar cane juice that has only the water removed and is milled to a powder. Grown without pesticides and used as a substitute for white or brown sugar. Light brown in color.

Sweet Potato Noodles (Kuzu-Kiri): Thin spaghetti-like noodles made of sweet potato starch and kuzu starch from the Japanese Kuzu bush. Commonly used in Oriental cooking.

Tahini: A thick paste made from ground sesame seeds and used like peanut butter.

Tapioca Starch: A preparation of cassava starch processed into granular flakes, pellets or flour. It can be used as a thickening agent in liquids.

Teff Flour: A grain that originated in Ethiopia. Contains more minerals and calcium than wheat or barley. Pancakes, waffles, and pastries can be made using teff without the addition of other flours. Gluten-free, it is a good wheat substitute. Available in white (ivory), brown, or red.

Tofu: A soybean product made from soybean curd. It is available in a soft, medium or a firm consistency. The soft cakes are generally used for sauces, while the firmer cakes may be used to replace meats in vegetarian dishes. Also used as a cottage cheese substitute.

Yogurt: A lactic fermentation of milk. A bacterial culture is used to bring about the fermentation. It comes in a variety of sizes, flavors and brands, many with a low butterfat content. It has many varied uses.

Yogurt Cheese: Can be made following the simple directions in this book. Used as a spread, in cooking, and as a substitute for cream cheese.

SECTION TWO

MEATLESS HAMBURGERS & CHOPPED LIVER • UNPUMPKIN PIE • EGG-FREE MAYO • SUGAR-FREE APPLE PIE • YEAST-FREE BREADSTICKS • MILK-FREE CREAMED SOUP • WHEAT-FREE PIZZA QUICHE • UNCOFFEE •

SUBSTITUTIONS ...
"PRESTO CHANGE-O"

This is it—the substitutions you always wanted to know about, but never dreamed of finding all in one place!

In the back of the book you will find a Brand Name Product Guide. This guide will help you locate the particular brand name products that I recommend. I have found these items to be nutritious, and tasty, yet less chemically contaminated. As you begin to read labels and know what additives you wish to avoid you can take advantage of the many new products that are just as good.

Now just turn the pages to a new adventure in cooking.

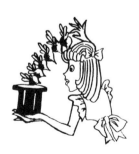

❤ SUBSTITUTION INDEX

AGAR-AGAR

Substitution:

Unflavored gelatin
1 tablespoon gelatin to jell two cups liquid

Soften 1 tablespoon gelatin in 1/2 cup cold liquid for 1 minute. Then add 1 1/2 cups of boiling liquid stirring to dissolve. Add sweetener if desired. Pour in mold and chill. May add 1 cup sliced fruit before chilling.

Note: High in calcium and magnesium, low in fat and calories. Be aware that agar-agar contains iodine; if you are sensitive use gelatin.

ARROWROOT FLOUR (STARCH)

Substitutions:

2 1/2 teaspoons arrowroot flour	= 1 tablespoon corn starch
	= 1/2 tablespoon potato starch
	= 1/2 tablespoon tapioca starch

Tapioca starch is especially good for thickening fruit juices.

BAKING POWDER

Substitutions:

Recipe No. 1

For 1 teaspoon baking powder
- 1/2   teaspoon cream of tartar
- 1/4   teaspoon baking soda

Recipe No. 2

Blend well and store in covered jar:
- 3/4   cup cream of tartar
- 9   tablespoons baking soda
- 6   tablespoons potato starch

Recipe No. 3

Blend well and store in covered jar:
- 2   parts arrowroot starch
- 1   part baking soda
- 1   part cream of tartar

Note: Baking powder usually contains corn starch and aluminum. Rumford brand baking powder is aluminum-free but contains cornstarch.

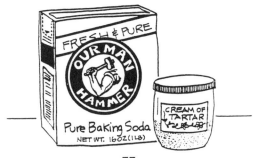

BISCUIT MIX

Commercial biscuit mixes usually contain baking powder, aluminum and corn.

Substitutions: For 1 cup biscuit mix

    1   cup kamut or unbleached white flour

    1 1/2 teaspoons baking powder substitute (see p. 33)

    1/2 teaspoon sea salt

    1   tablespoon organic ghee

Mix together well.

BOUILLON CUBES

Bouillon cubes may contain milk, wheat, corn or egg, MSG, and an excessive amount of salt.

Substitutions: For 1 bouillon cube

    1   tablespoon brewer's yeast (flakes or powder)

    1   tablespoon soy sauce

Most soy sauce contains wheat; however EDEN brand *Tamari* is wheat free. Be aware that low sodium soy sauce often contains added alcohol.

Barley Miso, another substitute for bouillon is traditionally made from soybeans, barley, water, and sea salt. Barley Miso has the highest mineral content of all misos. It is also apt to contain an excessive amount of salt—from 410 mg to 580 mg per tablespoon.

White and Red Misos, traditionally contain polished brown rice and soybeans.

Herb broth powders make good bouillon substitutes. One such powder available at health food stores is Dr. Bronner's Mineral Bouillon.

Bragg™ Liquid Aminos, also available in health food stores, are packaged in a convenient squeeze bottle you can place on the table and use as needed.

Defatted, undiluted beef or chicken drippings may also be frozen in ice cube trays and substituted as needed. To defat drippings, merely put drippings in refrigerator until the broth gels and you can see the fat on the surface. Skim off the fat and freeze the remaining drippings.

BREADSTUFFS

❤ BREADCRUMBS

Commercial breadcrumbs usually contain enriched, bleached white flour, hydrogenated vegetable oils, additives, and preservatives.

Substitutions that are wheat and gluten free:

> Crushed rice cereal
> Crushed potato chips, unsalted
> Crushed rye crisp crackers
> Crushed brown rice crackers
> Any dried 100% rice bread, grated

Substitutions that are not wheat and gluten free:

> Any dried 100% rye bread, grated
> Any dried whole wheat or rye Essene bread
> Crushed whole wheat matzoh crackers

Note: If not gluten or wheat sensitive, Jacklyn organic whole wheat additive-free breadcrumbs are available at health food stores.

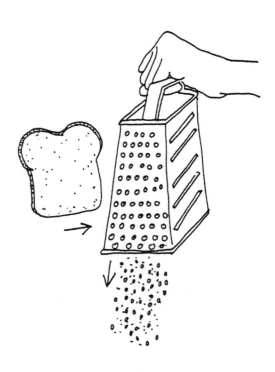

❤ MOCK GRAHAM CRACKERS (wheat and gluten-free)

- 1   cup teff flour
- 1/2   cup amaranth flour
- 3   teaspoons aluminum-free baking powder (see page 33)
- 1/4   teaspoon sea salt
- 1/2   cup sesame seed oil
- 6   tablespoons 100% maple syrup
- 2   well beaten egg whites

Combine first four ingredients in a large bowl and mix well. Mix oil with syrup and stir into flour mixture. Add egg whites and blend well. Form dough into a ball. Using 1/2 of the dough at a time, roll between 2 pieces of waxed paper till just under 1/4" thick (the thinner the cracker, the crispier). Discard top piece of waxed paper and cut the dough into rectangles using a pizza cutter. Carefully slide a metal spatula under each rectangle while gently pushing the rectangle onto the spatula, using the index finger of your other hand, and place onto a greased cookie sheet. Bake in preheated 375° oven for approximately 10 minutes or until edges of crackers are brown.

Can be crumbled and used as graham cracker crumbs.

For chocolate graham crackers substitute carob flour for amaranth and add an additional 3 tablespoons maple syrup.

♥ CRACKERS, WHITE FLOUR

Most commercial crackers contain refined, enriched white flour, hydrogenated vegetable oil, artificial flavoring, and preservatives.

Substitutions:

GLUTEN FREE:

> *Hol-Grain* brown rice crackers
> Most rice cakes and brown rice cakes
> *Health Valley* rice bran crackers
> *Edward & Sons* brown rice snaps
> *Wasa* rye crackers

YEAST-FREE:

> *Floridor* rye crisp
> *Ka·me* rice wafers
> *Hol-Grain* brown rice thins
> *Garden of Eatin'* organic whole wheat tortillas, toasted in the toaster oven
> Whole wheat matzoh crackers

YEASTED:

> *Kavli* Norwegian flatbread

❤ CROUTONS

Make your own from the substitution that is right for you:

> Any 100% rye, 100% whole wheat, or 100% rice bread (yeasted or unyeasted) make delicious croutons. Just cube, toss in extra virgin olive oil, and place on cookie sheet in 250° oven for about 45 minutes until crisp. Optional seasonings: garlic powder, dill, basil, oregano.

BUTTER

Unless you are dairy sensitive, a little butter in the context of a low fat diet can do no harm. Avoid hydrogenated (hardened) fats and oils such as margarine, shortenings, and factory-produced foods to which these modified oils and fats have been added. They are difficult to digest and interfere with normal cell metabolism. Recent research shows that these trans fatty acids can cause heart disease and cancer.

❤ BETTER BUTTERS

Ghee, or clarified butter, which has been used in India and in the Middle East for centuries, is becoming popular in America. Ghee is made from cow's milk, yet is virtually lactose free, since the milk solids are removed. Ghee does not turn rancid, nor does it bubble, smoke or burn. You can prepare it easily in your own kitchen using the following recipe.

❤ GHEE

Utensils you will need:

> heavy saucepan
> cheesecloth
> ladle
> clean glass jar or crock with tight-fitting lid
> fine mesh wire skimmer

Place butter in a saucepan. Allow the butter to melt, either on top of the stove or in the oven. Stir occasionally, and bring the butter to a slow boil. When a layer of foam covers the surface, lower the heat and continue to cook undisturbed for about 1 hour, on top of the stove, or slightly longer (up to 1 1/2 hours) in the oven. By then the butter will have separated. Under the layer of solid white surface foam will be amber-colored clarified butter (ghee) and at the bottom of the saucepan there will be some sediment. The water has evaporated and the milk solids have separated from the original butter.

Without shaking the saucepan, use the fine

mesh wire skimmer to carefully skim off as much foam as you can from the surface. Then strain the clear liquid ghee through several thicknesses of cheesecloth to remove the remaining foam. Ladle the clarified ghee into the clean glass jar or crock and seal tightly. Refrigerate or freeze.

For seasoned ghee, add your choice of herb when you melt the butter. Strain it out of the ghee when you pour it through the cheesecloth.

Organic ghee is also available at most health food stores.

If avoiding butter mainly because of its high cholesterol and saturated fat, try using blended butter. 1/4 pound of butter is turned into 2/3 pound.

❤ BLENDED BUTTER

1	organic egg white
2	tablespoons organic non-fat milk powder
2/3	cup high-oleic safflower oil
1/4	pound organic butter, room temperature

Combine milk powder and egg white. Let set 5 minutes. Add oil slowly, beating well with each addition. Add softened butter and blend until smooth. Store in covered dish in refrigerator.

Caution: Salmonella contamination is always a possibility when eating uncooked eggs.

Add equal parts of softened organic butter or organic ghee to high-oleic safflower oil in blender and blend until smooth. This butter melts more rapidly than Blended Butter, but it is great on toast and for sautéing. Keep in freezer until serving time to ensure firmness.

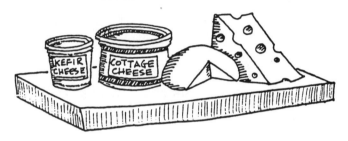

CHEESE—THE TWO-EDGED SWORD

Cheese is an excellent source of complete protein and it is also easy to digest; however, if you are mold sensitive, you should eat cheese with great caution as cheese grows mold and/or yeast. Cottage cheese, cream cheese, Romano cheese, and American tend to be yeast-free, but do contain mold, as do all other cheeses.

When you are shopping for cheese, pick out uncolored, unsalted cheese. There is no such thing as "natural" cheese, but there are many "unadulterated" cheeses available.

If your concern is pesticide residues, choose low-fat or organic milk cheeses, as pesticides are stored in the fat cells of the milk.

If you wish a non-dairy alternative, there are many styles of soy-based cheeses to choose from. They are not fat-free, however, so be sure to read the labels. The average fat content in a one ounce serving is approximately five grams. Many brands contain calcium caseinate, a milk protein, with only the lactose removed. Others are labeled 100 percent dairy free. Some alternatives are made using organic tofu and organic soy milk, while others are not organic. They all have a host of ingredients listed on the label. Always check for sodium content as it varies considerably from one style to the next.

Health food stores carry a wide array of these look- and taste-alikes that can be used in any way real cheese is used. Some of the types available are: mozzarella, cheddar, Parmesan, American, and Monterey Jack. Some brands offer grated, shredded, or sliced, as well as bulk. When purchasing a shredded style use it rather quickly, as it tends to form a solid mass within a week or so. Always keep refrigerated, or freeze if you intend to keep it for more than two weeks.

♥ COTTAGE CHEESE

Substitution:

> Tofu pressed and crumbled. Use as you
> would use cottage cheese in equal
> proportions.

Note: Before using tofu slice it and press between
layers of cloth or paper toweling to remove some
of the excess moisture. The weight of a breadboard
placed on top of the tofu will also help remove
moisture. To store unused portions, put back in
the refrigerator covered with fresh water. If you
change water often, it will keep up to two weeks.

Unflavored tofu is an excellent substitute for
cheese. And "reduced fat" tofu is available for fat
gram counters. Tofu is a complete protein and a
good source of iron, phosphorus and other nutrients. It adds nutrition to stews, soups, and desserts.
Tofu can be simmered, steamed, fried, marinated,
baked, or puréed. By itself it is very bland, but it
absorbs flavors readily. This allows you to season
tofu to suit your taste.

Unflavored tofu is pasty white in color, has the
consistency of a firm custard, and is usually packaged in brick form.

Extra firm style: Use as meat replacement. Cut in
cubes in stir-fry.

Regular style: Use crumbled as a cottage cheese replacement or in casseroles as a meat replacement.

Soft style: Use for sauces, gravies, desserts.

Tofu is also sold dried, fried, marinated or aged.

❤ CREAM CHEESE

Substitutions that are **not** *dairy-free:*

> Kefir cheese
> Yogurt cheese

Turn 1 pint of organic fat-free plain yogurt into a triple layer of cheesecloth about 1 square foot in size. Draw all corners of cloth up together and secure with a string or rubber band and attach to sink faucet and let hang about 8 hours until consistency of cream cheese. Untie and remove cloth and store yogurt cheese in covered container in refrigerator. Keeps about 1 week.

Substitutions that **are** *dairy free:*

Any dairy-free yogurt from health food stores can be turned into cheese using the same method. "Cream cheese style" non-dairy alternatives are available at health food stores.

CHOCOLATE

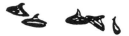

Chocolate is a highly allergenic food. It contains caffeine, oxalic acid, which interferes with calcium assimilation, and is high in fat. Carob, a chocolate alternative, is lower in fat, less bitter than chocolate, caffeine-free and high in vitamins and minerals.

❤ CHOCOLATE CHIPS

Substitution:

Equal amounts carob chips

Caution: Most carob chips contain sweeteners, fats, and milk products. However, *Sunspire* carob chips and chocolate chips are available dairy-free, sweetened or unsweetened.

❤ CHOCOLATE CHIPS, MELTED

Substitution: For 6 ounces chocolate chips:

- 1/2 cup carob powder
- 3/4 cup hot water
- 3 tablespoons 100 percent maple syrup
  Optional: Up to 2 tablespoons organic ghee

Heat in double boiler to spreading consistency.

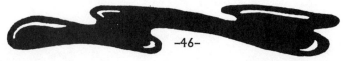

♥ CHOCOLATE PUDDING

Substitution:

   3   cups nut milk (see milk substitutions)
   6   tablespoons carob powder
   1/2 cup + 1 tablespoon maple syrup granules
   1/4 cup tapioca starch
   1   tablespoon ghee

In saucepan, mix tapioca starch, maple syrup granules and carob. Add nut milk gradually, continuously stirring while bringing mixture to a boil. Remove from heat. Add butter, and boil one minute longer, stirring until smooth and shiny.
MAKES 4 SERVINGS

Imagine Foods Non-dairy Dream Pudding is made with carob. The only non-dairy chocolate pudding substitute I have been able to find, it is available in health food stores.

❤ CHOCOLATE SYRUP

Substitution: Carob Syrup

- 1/2   cup carob powder
- 1/2   cup 100% maple syrup
- 1/3   cup organic ghee
- 1/3   cup raw cashew milk (see milk substitutions)
- 1/3   cup water

Place all ingredients in blender except the ghee. Blend and transfer to saucepan and bring to a boil, stirring constantly. Boil 1 minute. Remove from heat and beat in ghee until mixture is smooth and glossy. Keeps well refrigerated. YIELD: 1 1/2 CUPS

❤ UNSWEETENED CHOCOLATE

Substitution: For 1 ounce unsweetened chocolate:

- 3   tablespoons carob powder
- 1 1/2 tablespoons high-oleic safflower oil or 2 tablespoons water

Heat in top of double boiler and blend until smooth.

❤ UNSWEETENED COCOA

Substitution:

Equal amounts carob powder

CINNAMON

Processed cinnamon sold commercially may contain corn or wheat fillers. Whole cinnamon sticks may be purchased and ground to a powder in the blender.

Substitution:

Equal amounts coriander alone or

3   parts coriander
1   part anise seed
1/2 part ground sassafras

Note: Frontier Herbs cinnamon is 100 percent cinnamon. Available in most health food stores in glass jars.

COFFEE

Corn and corn sugars may be present in coffee, as well as caffeine.

❤ MOCK ICED COFFEE

1 1/3 cups low-fat milk or soy beverage
2/3 cup prune juice
1   egg
1   teaspoon lemon juice
2   ice cubes

Mix all together in blender until ice is completely melted. Serve immediately.

Substitutions available in health food stores:

Bambu: A combination of chicory, figs, wheat, barley, and acorns.

Roastaroma: A blend of roasted barley, malt, chicory root, carob, dandelion root, cinnamon, allspice, ginger and Chinese star anise. It tastes surprisingly like coffee and is caffeine free.

Cafix: A blend of malt, chicory, barley, rye, beet root and figs.

Yannoh: Organically grown cereal grain substitute containing barley, rye, malted barley, chicory, acorns (the acorns are not organically grown).

Café Altura: An organically-grown coffee, naturally low in caffeine.

Dacopa: 100 percent roasted dahlia syrup. Can be mixed with water or milk, hot or cold.

CORN OIL

Substitutions:

Organic, extra virgin olive oil
Peanut oil
High-oleic sunflower oil
High-oleic safflower oil
Organic ghee
Organic unrefined canola oil

CORN STARCH

Substitutions: For 1 tablespoon corn starch

2 1/2 teaspoons arrowroot starch
2 tablespoons whole wheat pastry flour
1/2 tablespoon potato starch
2 tablespoons kamut flour

Caution: Do not use arrowroot starch in a recipe that has to be rewarmed as it loses its thickening capacity.

CORN SYRUP

Substitutions in equal proportions:

Molasses
Sorghum
Honey
Maple syrup
Barley malt syrup plus 1/3 cup more
Brown rice syrup
Fruitsource™ liquid sweetener

CREAM

❤ SOUR CREAM

Substitutions that are not *dairy free:*

In equal parts:
Cow's milk fat-free yogurt
Goat's milk yogurt

♥ MOCK SOUR CREAM

    1   pint large-curd, low fat cottage cheese
    1/4–1/2 cup non-fat milk
    2   tablespoons lemon juice

Run cold water over cheese that has been placed in a strainer. When water runs clear let set to drain at least 5 minutes. Pour the curds into blender with milk and lemon juice and whir until smooth.

♥ KEFIR CHEESE (available in health food stores)

    Honey to taste, optional

Non-dairy substitution:

    Soy Yogurt—Many brands are available at health food stores.

♥ SWEET CREAM

Non-dairy substitution:

RECIPE NO. 1

Use in equal proportions:
    1   lightly poached egg or 1 raw egg yolk
    2   tablespoons high-oleic safflower oil
    1–2 tablespoons honey
    lemon juice to taste

Mix all ingredients in blender until smooth. If too thick, a little water may be added. Refrigerate if necessary to thicken. Cannot be used in recipes calling for large amounts of cream.

Caution: Salmonella contamination is always a possibility when eating undercooked eggs.

RECIPE NO. 2

Blend well-drained firm or silken tofu (see page 44) with brown rice syrup to taste in food processor.

❤ WHIPPING CREAM

Substitution that is not *dairy-free:*

RECIPE NO. 1

Whipped Evaporated Milk

For the cholesterol and calorie conscious. Add a dash of vanilla or other flavoring to disguise the canned milk flavor. Not as stiff as Recipe No. 2.

Dairy-free substitutions:

RECIPE NO. 2

SOY WHIPPING "CREAM"

2	egg whites
1	cup ice water
1	cup powdered soy beverage
2	teaspoons vanilla
2	tablespoons *Ohsawa* brown rice syrup powder (optional)

Chill beaters and bowl 1/2 hour. Beat 2 egg whites in chilled bowl until almost firm, then add ice water and powdered soy, and beat until stiff. Add vanilla and powdered syrup at the same time. Store in refrigerator until ready for use.

Caution: Salmonella contamination is always a possibility when eating raw eggs.

RECIPE NO. 3

TOFU WHIPPING "CREAM"
6	ounces drained tofu (see page 44)
1	tablespoon honey
1	teaspoon vanilla

Blend all ingredients in blender until smooth. Will be thick but not stiff.

EGGS

Note: If you are allergic to eggs or dairy, read the label before using a commercial egg substitute. They usually contain egg whites and non-fat milk solids.

Substitutions: As a binder for meat and vegetable dishes:

1 egg = 1 1/2 tablespoons high-oleic safflower oil
        1 1/2 tablespoons carbonated spring water
        1 teaspoon potato starch, or

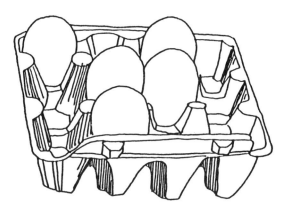

1 teaspoon non-aluminum baking powder
(see page 33). Use 1 teaspoon baking powder
for each egg up to two eggs, if recipe already
calls for oil.

As a binder in custard:

1 egg = 1 tablespoon potato starch or corn starch
1 tablespoon gelatin to 2 cups of non-fat milk

First, soak gelatin in 1/4 cup cold milk. Heat
remaining milk and combine. Set aside to thicken,
then beat until light and bubbly. Follow pudding
directions for additional flavorings.

As a leavener in baking:

1 egg = 2 tablespoons carbonated spring water and
2 teaspoons non-aluminum baking powder

Beat an extra minute to incorporate air into mix.
Never try to replace more than two eggs. Some-

times carbonated spring water alone works in pan-cakes and muffins.

As a binder and leavener for cookies:

1 egg = 3 tablespoons pureed fruit, such as bananas or apricots

Or mix together well: 2 parts arrowroot powder, 1 part tapioca flour, 1 part slippery elm powder.

1 egg = 1 tablespoon above dry mix plus 1–2 table-spoons carbonated water

As a binder and leavener (not for use in cookies):

1 egg = 1 1/2 tablespoons high-oleic safflower oil
1 1/2 tablespoons carbonated spring water
2 tablespoons non-aluminum baking powder (see page 38)

= 1 tablespoon liquid lecithin or 1 tablespoon lecithin granules with 2 tablespoons water

= 1 tablespoon garbanzo flour with 1 table-spoon oil (some leavening)

= 1 banana (as a binder)

= 2 tablespoons flaxseed mix
Blend 3 cups water with 1 cup ground flax-seeds in blender until smooth. Store in cov-ered jar in refrigerator.

= 3 tablespoons apricot mix
Soak 1/2 pound sun-dried apricots in water for 8 hours. Blend and strain. Store in closed jar in refrigerator.

= 1 teaspoon *Ener-G Egg Replacer* (does not contain egg white but does contain milk solids) combined with 2 tablespoons water.

Caution: If you are allergic to eggs or milk, read the labels on commercial egg substitutes, as they often contain egg white and nonfat milk solids.

❤ EGG WHITES

1 egg white = 2¹/4 teaspoons skim milk powder or soy beverage powder + 2 teaspoons high-oleic safflower oil, blended together in a food processor or blender

❤ EGG YOLK

Substitutions: For leavening

1 egg yolk = ¹/2 teaspoon non-aluminum baking powder
= 2 tablespoons soy flour

For binding:

1 egg yolk = 2 tablespoons of the following mixture: Using 1 part soy flour plus 2 parts water, mix in blender until thickened and double boil 1 hour. Beat in 2 tablespoons of high-oleic oil for each cup of flour mix. Place in covered jar in refrigerator.

GARLIC POWDER AND GARLIC SALT

Substitution:

> If your main concern is chemicals, use
> minced organic whole garlic, or organic gar-
> lic oil, which may be purchased as a food
> supplement in capsule form.

GELATIN (JELL-O)

Gelatin is an animal product that is used to jell
fruit juices, fruit pies and other liquids.

Substitution:

> Agar-agar (do not use if iodine sensitive)
> 2 tablespoons agar-agar jells 3 1/2 cups liquid

Soften agar-agar in 1 cup of liquid for 1 minute. Then
add to hot liquid and boil for 2 minutes. Let cool before
adding fruit. May add sweetener if desired.

Note: Kuzu root starch—prepare as directed on
package. If potato allergic, purchase 100 percent
Kuzu root to avoid the addition of potato starch.

ICE CREAM

There are many health reasons for avoiding commercial ice creams. Not only are they high in sugar and fat but they contain the same chemical additives that are used in paint remover, anti-freeze, pesticides, plastic, rubber, leather cleaner and paint solvents.

I have listed the more chemical-free health food store alternatives, including dairy-free and sugar-free brands, plus several very pleasing homemade substitutions.

Häagen-Dazs, Ben and Jerry's and *Breyer's* are three national brands that are additive free. They are sweetened with honey/cane sugar or maple syrup. Their labels are explicit.

❤ BASIC ICE CREAM MIX

    1   cup heavy cream
    1³/4 cups low fat milk
    1¹/4 cups 100% maple syrup

For Maple Walnut Ice Cream add 3/4 cup organic chopped walnuts.

For Strawberry Ice Cream, add 2 pints of freshly washed hulled and split berries and replace maple syrup (for sugar-free) with 1 1/2 jars fruit juice sweetened strawberry spreadable fruit preserves. Or use peaches with peach preserves, etc.

If you don't have an ice cream maker, this mixture may be blended in a blender, then placed in a bowl in the freezer until firm. Remove and whip with electric beaters and refreeze. Thaw about 5 to 10 minutes before serving.

YIELD: APPROXIMATELY 1 1/2 PINTS

Lowfat substitution:

FROZEN YOGURT. Choose those with active cultures. Made from lowfat milk, yogurt, sugar, fruit, natural flavorings and gelatin (some contain chemicals). Fruit juice sweetened brands are also available.

Dairy-free substitutions:

ICE BEAN is soy based, honey sweetened and dairy free.

RICE DREAM is rice-based, sweetened with maple syrup and is soy and dairy-free.

Sorbets and Italian Ices: Contain no milk, cream, or fat. Contain fruit, water, and a large percentage of sugar. Sugar-free versions are found in health food stores.

VITARI is 100% fruit with no fat, no lactose, no added sugar. Fruit only.

❤ CREAMSICLES

Substitutions:

Mix plain organic fat-free yogurt with fruit juice to taste and freeze.

CAROB

> 1 cup organic fat-free yogurt
> 1/4 cup carob powder
> 1/4 cup 100% maple syrup

Mix in blender and freeze, using same method as popsicles, below.

For non-diary, use soy yogurt or silken tofu to replace yogurt.

❤ POPSICLES

Substitutions:

Freeze unsweetened fruit juice in purchased molds or in 3 ounce paper cups, placing a stick in the center of each just before freezing takes place. To eat, just peel away cup. You can add a small amount of dissolved gelatin to liquid to make the popsicles less drippy.

Puréed fresh or dried fruit, which has first been soaked in hot water, then drained, may be frozen in the same manner; use puréed *fresh* fruit if mold sensitive.

❤ SHERBET

Substitutions:

1 1/4 cups fruit juice sweetened spreadable fruit preserves or

1 cup fresh berries with 1/2 cup 100% maple syrup

2 cups water

2 egg whites, stiffly beaten (optional)

In blender, mix preserves and water. Spoon into bowl and freeze until firm. Remove from freezer and, using electric mixer, mix with egg whites until light and airy. Serve immediately. SERVES 4–6

Organic fruit sorbets are available at health food stores.

ICINGS

Most cake frostings are made from exorbitant amounts of sugar laden with chemical colorings and flavorings, some of which are cancer-causing. There is an ongoing debate over the safety of many of these pigments. May also contain other questionable ingredients.

Substitutions:

❤ CAROB BUTTERCREAM FROSTING

    1/2 cup + tablespoon 100% maple syrup or
         brown rice syrup powder
    8   tablespoons organic butter or soy marga-
         rine, softened
    3/4 cup carob powder

Place butter and syrup in bowl and blend together well. Add carob powder, a little at a time, beating well after each addition. Continue beating by hand until smooth.

Beat in organic non-fat milk powder or powdered soy beverage if a thicker frosting is desired.

YIELD: 1 HEAPING CUP

Note: Frosting becomes quite firm when chilled due to butter content.

❤ VANILLA DRIZZLE

    3   *tablespoons low-fat rice milk*
    1   *tablespoon honey*
    1/2 *teaspoon vanilla*
    3/4 *teaspoon arrowroot powder*

Heat 2 tablespoons of rice milk with honey and vanilla in saucepan. Dissolve arrowroot powder in

1 tablespoon of milk and add to warm mixture. Continue stirring and heating until thickened and drizzle over cupcakes, etc.

Do not rewarm—arrowroot will lose its thickening capacity.

To color Vanilla Drizzle, try any of the following in small amounts:

> *red* — beet or red fruit juice
> *orange* — orange, papaya, or carrot juice
> *green* — wheat grass (powdered) or parsley juice
> *blue* — blueberry juice

MAPLE-ONLY FROSTING

> 1 cup of 100% maple syrup granules powdered in blender
> 4 teaspoons cold water

Blend and spread on cakes or cookies; or use Maple Butter, a ready-to-spread whipped maple syrup.

JAMS

Most commercial jams contain an excess of refined sugars, corn sweeteners, and pesticides. However, there are many organic fruit juice sweetened jams available in health food stores.

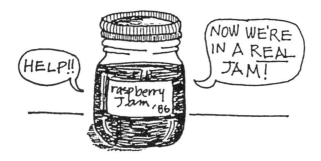

Substitutions:

❤ RASPBERRY JAM (or any fresh fruit)

> 1   *cup fresh raspberries*
> 1   *tablespoon honey, or more to taste*

Wash, drain and blend berries with honey in blender. Pour in saucepan and bring to a boil. Turn to low and simmer, stirring frequently, until mixture reaches desired thickness.

YIELD: APPROXIMATELY 1/3 CUP

❤ DRIED FRUIT PRESERVES

> 8   *ounces dried fruit*
> 2   *tablespoons lemon juice*
>   *honey, to taste*

Chop fruit fine and stir in lemon juice. Top with honey and place in a covered bowl for 4 to 5 days until very soft. Place in jar in refrigerator, to store.

YIELD: APROXIMATELY 2 CUPS

KETCHUP

Ketchup contains white sugar (may or may not be corn based) and contains yeast due to the nature of its preparation.

Substitution:

❤ KETCHUP QUICKIE

  8   tomatoes
  1/4 cup maple sugar granules or powdered brown rice syrup
  1   teaspoon sea salt
       lemon juice, to taste
       minced onion, to taste (optional)

Parboil tomatoes for 10 minutes to soften skins and using the back of a spoon, press the tomatoes through a sieve into a saucepan. Discard the remaining seeds and skin. Add remaining ingredients and cook, uncovered, on simmer until sauce is desired thickness (about 1 to 1 1/2 hours). Keep well refrigerated in a covered glass jar. YIELD: 2 CUPS

LEMON JUICE CONCENTRATE

Commercial lemon juice concentrate may contain sodium benzoate and sodium bisulfite as preservatives. Sodium bisulfite is a suspected mutagen, but it is still regarded as safe at the present levels of use as a preservative. It remains on the "Generally Regarded As Safe" list with restrictions on the amounts that can be added to foods.

Commercial lemons, as well as lemon concentrate contain pesticide residues. As a precaution, when making lemon zest, always use organic lemons.

Substitutions:

Organic lemonade concentrate or fresh squeezed organic lemons, in equal proportions, in recipes.

Lemonade Substitution:

If allergic to citrus, remove the citric acid powder from one or more vitamin C capsules. Add water and honey to taste. Shake to blend. Add crushed ice if desired.

MAYONNAISE

May or may not contain corn oil. Contains yeast by the nature of its manufacture. Also contains artificial stabilizers.

Substitutions:

❤ MAYODELICIOUS (corn, yeast, dairy-free)

   3/4 cup plain soy yogurt
   1   green onion, chopped
   1   tablespoon fruit juice sweetened peach
        spreadable fruit preserves
        dry mustard and sea salt, to taste

❤ QUICK MAYO (corn-free, but *not* yeast or dairy-free)

Mix *Walnut Acres No-Yolk Mayonnaise Dressing* (contains egg whites) into kefir cheese until desired flavor is reached. Add honey, to taste, if desired. Delicious in egg salad or potato salad.

❤ SOY MAYO (corn, yeast, dairy-free)

   3   tablespoons soy milk powder
   1/2 cup water
   1   cup high-oleic safflower oil
   1   tablespoon 100% maple syrup
   1   teaspoon sea salt
   1   green onion, chopped fine, bulb only
   1/4 cup lemon juice

Place first two ingredients in blender and blend until well mixed (a few seconds). Add the maple syrup, sea salt, and green onion. Add oil next, and continue blending on low until mixture is thick. Add lemon juice. Refrigerate in covered jar.

YIELD: APPROXIMATELY 1 1/2 CUPS

MERINGUE

Egg-free substitution:

> 5   tablespoons ground flaxseeds and 5 cups cold water

Soak flaxseeds in water for an hour. Simmer 20 minutes and then strain. Set in refrigerator to cool. Beat as you would egg whites.

Use only as a topping in recipes requiring no further cooking. It will not hold up under heat.

MILK, COW'S

Aside from being allergic to milk protein or lacking the ability to digest it (lactose intolerance), there are other reasons to be wary of drinking cow's milk. Hormone, pesticide, and antibiotic residues sporadically show up in milk samples. Since pesticides collect in animal fat cells, there are apt to be more pesticide residues in whole milk products. And milk from organically raised cows is not always available.

Another potential problem with commercial milk is that it has been pasteurized and homogenized.

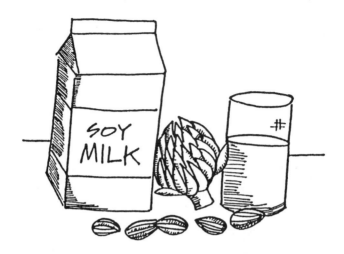

Once processed, the superb nutritional value of the raw milk has been diminished. The high heat during pasteurization is responsible. And a more recent suspicion, that the homogenization process causes biological changes in the fat structure of milk, may be the cause of circulatory problems in some people. While awaiting further research, it would be prudent to try some of the many good alternatives to high fat and homogenized milk products.

Goat's milk is apt to be less contaminated than cow's milk, as it is produced on smaller farms where sanitation is less of a problem. And although goat's milk is more easily digested than cow's milk, the fat content of goat's milk is its disadvantage. It has a slightly higher fat content than whole cow's milk.

The two most popular nondairy alternatives to

milk are soy-based beverages and rice-based beverages. Some are totally organic, while others have one or two organic ingredients in them. And like milk, you can have your choice of approximately 2 grams of fat per 8 ounce serving (the lite style) or approximately 7 grams of fat, per 8 ounce serving (the regular style). Almond, chocolate, vanilla, and carob are the most popular flavors to choose from. And the ingredients change with each flavor and brand.

The soy beverages generally contain water, soybeans, malted cereal extracts, barley malt and corn. So gluten intolerants and corn allergics beware. However, *Pacific Foods Organic Soy Beverage* does not contain any sweeteners and would be acceptable for gluten intolerants.

The rice beverages generally contain water, brown rice, and high-oleic safflower oil.

I find the rice beverages taste the most like dairy milk and are excellent in cereals. My favorite brand is *Rice Dream Original Lite* because it is produced using organic brown rice, unrefined high-oleic safflower oil, and contains only 2 grams of fat per 8 ounce serving.

Caution: Soy and rice milks are not intended for use as infant formulas.

As a rule of thumb:

- **If gluten and dairy sensitive, use a rice beverage.**

- If rice and dairy sensitive, use a soy beverage.

- If soy and dairy sensitive, use a rice beverage.

- If chocolate and dairy sensitive, use a carob/soy or carob/rice beverage.

Notes: Rennet custards will coagulate only with cow's milk. Do not boil sauces or puddings made with soy milk as they will separate. Be careful to heat just to boiling. Baking with soy milk will be no problem. Nut milk thickens quickly on high heat.

❤ MILK

Quickie substitutions to prepare from scratch:

NOT DAIRY-FREE:

1 cup whole cow's milk	= 1 cup goat's milk, if lactalbumin is the only consideration
	= 6 tablespoons *Walnut Acres Organic Nonfat Milk Powder* (non-instant) plus 1 cup water, well blended

EASY DAIRY-FREE SUBSTITUTIONS:

1	cup fruit juice (good in cereal)
1	cup carbonated spring water (especially good in baking for additional leavening)

♥ BUTTERMILK OR SOUR MILK

Substitutions:

1   cup organic fat-free plain yogurt curdled with 1 tablespoon lemon juice (fresh if yeast is a concern) or the citric acid from 2 vitamin C capsules.

or

1   cup fat-free milk curdled with 1 tablespoon vinegar (or fresh lemon juice if yeast-sensitive)

DAIRY-FREE VERSION:

1   cup soft tofu blended with 1 tablespoon lemon juice and 1/2 teaspoon sea salt.

♥ CHOCOLATE MILK

There are many organic and non-organic carob and chocolate dairy-free milk substitutes available at health food stores. But you must read the labels if you are purchasing them for reasons other than just being dairy-free.

Substitutions:

Carob syrup (see page 48) added to your choice of milk or milk substitute, to taste.

CHOCO-DATE NUT MILK

1 1/2 cups cashew nut milk (see page 76)

3   tablespoons carob powder
5   cut-up dates
1   tablespoon peanut butter
      Dash of vanilla, optional

Blend together in blender and chill. YIELD: 2 CUPS

HOT CHOCOLATE

Simply heat either of the above recipes on low until desired temperature.

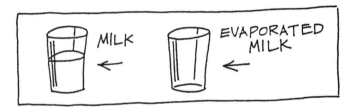

❤ EVAPORATED MILK

Substitutions:

> *Pacific Foods Soy Beverage* (no sweeteners and gluten-free)
>
> Use evaporated goat's milk if lactalbumin (curds and whey) is the only consideration.

❤ POWDERED MILK

Commercial powdered milk is subjected to high heat during manufacturing.

Substitutions:

> Equal amounts powdered soy beverage (if milk allergic)
>
> Equal amounts powdered yogurt
>
> Equal amounts goat's milk powder (if lact-albumin is the only consideration)

Note: If pesticide avoidance is your only reason for avoiding milk, look for organic, non-fat powdered milk in the health food store.

❤ SWEETENED CONDENSED MILK

Commercial brands may contain excessive amounts of refined sugar. Phenol lined cans may be a problem for chemically sensitive individuals.

Substitution:

1 cup = one cup of the following mixture:

> 1   cup organic nonfat dry milk (if dairy sensitive, use powdered soy beverage)
>
> 2/3 cup brown rice syrup powder
>
> 1/3 cup boiling water
>
> 1/4 cup organic ghee

Combine all ingredients in blender and blend until smooth.

❤ NUT MILK

- 1/2 cup raw cashews or peanuts
- 1 cup water
- 1 teaspoon *Ohsawa Brown Rice Syrup Powder*
  Cook's Vanilla Powder (in a dextrose sugar base, but containing no alcohol), optional

Grind nuts in nut grinder until pasty. Remove to blender. Add water and blend on high until smooth. Add powdered brown rice syrup and vanilla and blend for a few seconds more. Use cup for cup.

❤ SESAME SEED NUT MILK:

RECIPE #1

- 1 cup sesame seeds
- 2 cups water
- 1 1/2 teaspoons brown rice syrup

RECIPE #2

- 1 1/2 cups sesame seeds
- 1/4 cup currants or raisins
- 3 cups of water

Blend well, but don't strain. Excellent for use in puddings, on cereal, and for cooking and baking.

❤ ALMOND MILK

- 5 tablespoons blanched almonds or 6 tablespoons almond butter

1 cup water
1 teaspoon honey, or more to taste

Blend in blender till smooth or try *Ener-G Nutquick* almond milk powder (available in health food stores).

❤ POTATO WATER (for bread baking)

Boil 2 cups of chopped and peeled potatoes in 3 cups of water until soft, remove potatoes. YIELDS ABOUT 2 CUPS OF POTATO WATER. Make as needed.

❤ ARTICHOKE MILK
1/2 cup artichoke flour
2 cups water

Mix water and flour in saucepan with electric beater. Bring to a boil, then simmer for 20 minutes. Drink plain, or sweeten to taste.

❤ ZUCCHINI MILK
1 medium peeled zucchini
2 tablespoons 100% maple syrup or less, to taste
1 egg, beaten
Cook's Vanilla Powder optional

Whir zucchini in blender until smooth. Mix with syrup and heat on low. Add beaten egg to mixture and continue stirring until mixture thickens (8 to 10 minutes). If overcooked, it will separate. Put back in blender for a few seconds until smooth again. Chill and drink.

PANCAKE SYRUPS

Most commercial pancake syrups are blends of corn syrup, sugar, imitation maple flavoring, artificial coloring, and salt. Formaldehyde is used in the tapping process when removing the sap from the trees, unless you purchase organic, 100% pure maple syrup.

Substitutions:

> 100% apple butter, free of spices
> Mashed bananas
> *Fruitsource*™ liquid sweetener (rice and grape based)
> Homemade jams
> Organic 100% pure maple syrup
> *Knudson Pourable Fruit*

PASTA (White Flour)

Substitutions that are egg, milk and wheat free:

> Mung Bean Threads
> Sweet Potato Noodles (Kuzu-Kiri)
> Brown Rice Pasta

Corn Pasta

Tofu, sliced in thin strips (good in broth)

100% Buckwheat Noodles (Soba)

Rice Pasta, White

Quinoa Pasta (most quinoa pasta contains corn flour)

Spelt Pasta—a different type of wheat pasta that many wheat sensitive persons are able to tolerate.

PEANUT BUTTER

Most commercial peanut butter contains salt, artificial flavorings, hydrogenated vegetable oil, and various forms of sugar. Preservatives and emulsifiers are usually added.

Peanuts are susceptible to aflatoxin contamination. Aflatoxin is a carcinogen associated with liver cancer. The FDA suspects that raw peanuts have a greater level of contamination, as roasting may reduce aflatoxin levels. However, roasting does not kill an aflatoxin mold called *Aspergillus flavus.* It may be present in roasted peanuts, peanut butter, packaged nuts, and candy containing nuts. Peanut oils are free of the toxin because of the strong alkalis used in processing.

Two brands of peanut butter that are certified to be aflatoxin-free (and also free of chemical insecticides or fumigants) are: *Walnut Acres* and *Arrowhead Mills,* both available in health food stores.

♥ HOME-STYLE PEANUT BUTTER

Place any amount of dry or roasted peanuts in food processor, add 1 tablespoon of high-oleic safflower oil and begin to process. Drizzle in additional oil only as needed until desired consistency is reached. If you like crunchy peanut butter, simply stop the processor before nuts are completely ground. Store in a jar with a tight-fitting lid in the refrigerator.

Substitutions:

CASHEW BUTTER

Roast raw cashews for 15 minutes (or until lightly browned) in 350° oven. Grind in nut grinder until pasty. Add a touch of high-oleic vegetable oil, if needed to obtain a spreading consistency. Salt optional.

Almonds and pecans may be prepared the same way. Pecans will have a much richer taste.

Tahini is a thick paste that is made by grinding sesame seeds. It may be used as you would use peanut butter. Cashew butter, almond butter, and tahini are all available in health food stores.

PUMPKIN SEED NUT BUTTER

1   cup pumpkin seeds
1   tablespoon high-oleic vegetable oil (more if needed)
    sea salt or honey, optional

Blend in blender until smooth and store in closed jar in refrigerator.

Roasted soybeans may also be prepared in the same way.

PIE CRUST

When preparing pie crusts using non-gluten flours, I find them much easier to handle when rolling in a pie crust maker (a round zippered laminate bag). It makes the turning procedure much easier and you will have a perfect circle.

Wheat-free substitutions:

TEFF FLOUR PIE CRUST

1/4	cup high-oleic safflower oil
1/4	cup water
1	cup ivory teff flour
3	tablespoons powdered brown rice syrup

Beat oil and water together until frothy in a large bowl. Set aside. Combine flour with powdered syrup in a small bowl and mix well.

Combine the two mixtures in the larger bowl, and stir with a fork until mixture almost forms a dough ball. Pat together and roll out into an 11 inch circle between two pieces of waxed paper. Remove the top sheet of the paper and quickly turn dough into a lightly greased 9 inch pie plate.

Gently press together any tears. Flute the edges if desired. Prick bottom and sides with a fork.

Bake unfilled in a 375° oven for 15 minutes, or until lightly browned. Cool before filling.

COCONUT PIE CRUST

    3 1/2 ounces unsweetened coconut
    3   tablespoons organic ghee

Mix together and press into 8" pie plate. Bake in preheated 350° oven until browned on edges. Cool and fill.

NUT PIE CRUST

    1   cup ground pecans or almonds
    2   tablespoons 100% maple sugar granules
    1   tablespoon organic ghee

Mix together and press into an 8" pie plate. Use as is or place in 350° oven for about 10 minutes.

MERINGUE PIE CRUST NO. 1

    2   egg whites
    2   tablespoons 100% maple syrup
    1/4 teaspoon cream of tartar

Beat egg whites and cream of tartar until frothy. Beat in maple syrup, slowly, until the mixture forms stiff peaks. Spread in greased 9" pie plate, going up the sides as well. Place in preheated 350° F. oven, turning oven off immediately. Leave undisturbed in oven overnight.

MERINGUE PIE CRUST NO. 2

3   egg whites, room temperature
1/4 teaspoon cream of tartar
1/4 teaspoon sea salt
1/2 cup 100% maple syrup

Beat egg whites, salt and cream of tartar until soft peaks form. Slowly beat in maple syrup, until very stiff peaks form. Meringue will be shiny. Spread in lightly buttered 10" pie plate. Bake in preheated 275° F. oven for 45 minutes. Cool on wire rack.

THE SIMPLE SOYMAN

A superb frozen wheat-free, dairy-free pie crust with barley flour as the main ingredient is available in health food stores.

POTATO FLOUR (Starch)

Substitutions:
1/2 tablespoon
   potato starch = 1/2 tablespoon tapioca starch
               = 1 tablespoon corn starch
               = 1 tablespoon flour
               = 2 1/2 teaspoons arrowroot starch

Do not use arrowroot starch in a recipe that has to be rewarmed as it loses its thickening capacity. Tapioca starch is especially good for thickening fruit juices.

SALT

Most brands of table salt contain dextrose (sugar) and chemicals to ensure that they flow freely.

Substitutions:
Use, to taste, as you would table salt:

- **Kelp powder** (contains iodine and other essential nutrients)
- **Sea salt** (contains iodine and other essential nutrients)
- **Soy sauce** (also high in salt)
- *Bragg* **liquid aminos** (amino acids from vegetable protein)
- **Miso** (rich in protein, high in salt)

See also soy, page 84, bouillon, page 34

SAUCES AND GRAVIES

Substitutions:

CHINESE HOT SAUCE FOR EGG ROLLS

$1/2$ cup fruit juice sweetened pineapple spreadable fruit preserves

$1/2$ teaspoon (or more if you like it hot) brown mustard

or, preserves may be used alone for a sweeter sauce

CHINESE-STYLE BROWN GRAVY

3   tablespoons whole wheat pastry flour
1 1/2 tablespoons organic ghee
1/2 cup water
1/2 tablespoon *Bragg*™ liquid aminos

Brown flour in dry skillet on medium heat, constantly stirring, being careful not to burn (about 3 minutes). Reduce heat to simmer and blend in ghee until smooth. Add water slowly, stirring constantly until desired consistency is obtained. Add liquid aminos. Use in Chinese dishes as brown sauce or serve over mashed potatoes or stuffing. YIELD: APPROXIMATELY 1/2 CUP.

TOMATO SAUCE

1 1/2 cups stewed plum tomatoes
1   heaping tablespoon honey
1   heaping teaspoon arrowroot flour, optional
1/2 teaspoon sea salt
     minced garlic, to taste

Simmer tomatoes, honey and seasonings for 1/2 hour to thicken. Add arrowroot flour to a little water to make a paste and stir into sauce to thicken. (If you have time, omit arrowroot flour and simmer until sauce thickens naturally.) YIELD: 1 CUP.

❤ SOY SAUCE

(Also see salt, page 84; bouillon cubes, page 34)

Soy sauce is derived from soybeans and usually contains water, wheat, an excessive amount of salt, and 2.5% alcohol. The alcohol is generated during the fermentation process and serves as a preservative. It is not required to be listed on the label. Low sodium (approximately 160 mg per tablespoon) and naturally brewed soy sauce has additional alcohol added, and its presence is indicated on the label. Soy sauce contains anywhere from 500 mg to more than 2,000 mg of salt per tablespoon.

There are several types of soy sauce available, each containing slightly different ingredients. The following list should be of help if you are trying to avoid certain ingredients.

Shoyu: contains water, soybeans, wheat and salt.

Low Sodium Shoyu: same as above except double brewed, which removes some salt.

Tamari: wheat-free Shoyu sauce.

Substitutions:

RECIPE NO. 1

1/4 cup soy sauce =
3 tablespoons Worcestershire sauce and 1 tablespoon water.

Worcestershire sauce contains soy and various spices. If you are sensitive to soy, use:

RECIPE NO. 2

Very concentrated defatted beef broth with 3 parts
defatted beef drippings to 1 part water. Add sea salt
if desired. See page 35 for defatting instructions.

Or, *Bragg™ Liquid Aminos*—A non-fermented
vegetable protein (from soybeans) that is a salt-
free alternative. Use "a dash at a time." Available
in health food stores.

❤ WHITE CREAM SAUCE

    1   10 ounce package of frozen cauliflower,
         steamed
    1/4–1/2 cup clear defatted chicken or vegetable
         broth, warmed
    1/2 tablespoon high-oleic safflower oil
         salt and pepper to taste

Drain hot cauliflower well and place in blender.
On high speed, gradually add broth until thick and
creamy. Add oil and seasoning.

YIELD: APPROXIMATELY 1 CUP.

❤ TANGY CREAM SAUCE

    2   tablespoons organic ghee
    2   heaping teaspoons whole wheat pastry flour
    2/3 cup fat-free yogurt or soy yogurt
         sea salt and pepper to taste
         tarragon, optional

Melt ghee in saucepan and stir in flour until smooth. Bring to a boil. Remove from heat and stir in yogurt until well blended. Season and return to heat just long enough to reach serving temperature. YIELD: 2/3 CUP.

Note: High heat will destroy beneficial yogurt culture.

SHORTENING

See corn oil, page 50 and butter, page 39.

When substituting a liquid for a solid, reduce other liquids and bake a little longer at a lower temperature. One cup solid fat = 2/3 cup oil.

SODA POP

The sugar content alone is a good reason to avoid drinking soda. Soft drinks may contain 9 to 11 teaspoons of sugar per 12-ounce can. Other reasons to pass up soda pop are additives, artificial flavors, and colors. Phosphoric and citric acids are commonly used as flavor enhancers in soft drinks, and may cause teeth to dissolve over time. Unfortunately these changes are not easily visible until extensive damage has already been done. And sugar-free drinks have an even higher acid content.

Substitutions:

> 6 ounces carbonated spring water added to fresh or concentrated fruit juice to taste:
> > lime juice
> > lemon juice
> > apple juice
> > orange juice
> > apricot juice
> > raspberry juice
> > strawberry juice
> > grape juice
> > pineapple juice

Use brown rice syrup powder, for additional sweetening, if desired.

SPICES

If you are mold sensitive, be wary of using spices. Spices are also irradiated and laden with pesticides. If a spice has been irradiated, the label must say so. When storing spices, for optimum freshness, use a glass container with a tight-fitting lid. Metal containers with sifter tops will compromise the freshness of the contents.

Spices that are non-irradiated, organic, and packaged in glass jars are available in health food stores.

SWEET ROLLS

Substitutions:

CHEESE DANISH DELIGHT

1   whole wheat English Muffin cut in half, lightly toasted (or any whole grain toast)
crumbled tofu
fruit juice sweetened spreadable fruit preserves

Spread enough crumbled tofu on each muffin half to generously cover, and place a dollop of preserves in the center. Place in toaster oven to toast for a few minutes. Jam will spread, muffin will toast more, and tofu will be warm.

Serve as a quick breakfast when you are in a hurry.

For wheat-free diets use 100% rye Essene bread, toasted.

SWEETENERS

Some of the many names for sugar are: dextrose, fructose, lactose, sucrose, glucose, corn syrup, honey, molasses, maple sugar, brown sugar, raw sugar.

Honey raises blood sugar levels as much as sucrose. Refined sugars contain no nutritional value. I have only included maple syrup granules and maple syrup as substitutes because of their versatility and because of the nature of their manufacture.

Many of the larger maple syrup producers use form-aldehyde when extracting the sap from the tree. They may also add defoaming agents. But, if purchased as organic 100 percent pure, maple syrup is simply boiled-down maple tree sap.

I feel that a few words about low-caloric and non-caloric sweeteners are necessary because they are overused, leave our bodies confused, and should be avoided for optimal health.

Aspartame (*NutraSweet, Equal*) and saccharin (*Sweet 'n Low*) are the gruesome twosome most commonly used in foods. Several reports have suggested that aspartame may cause headaches, seizures, visual distortion and weight gain among other side effects, yet an estimated 100 million Americans use some form of it on a daily basis.

Aspartame is believed to have an adverse effect on children's brain functions. One component in aspartame, aspartic acid, an excitatory amino acid, is believed to be the cause of this damage. It acts as a neuro-exciter and at a high level, as a neurotoxin. It is especially damaging to the very young, according to Dr. John Olney, a professor of psychiatry at Washington University in St. Louis. He estimates that as few as two aspartame sweetened soda pops in a single day are enough to induce brain lesions. Olney further suggests that the brain damage may not be apparent until many years later; hence, cause and effect may go undetected.

Dieters who use aspartame to avoid the weight gain associated with sugar are fooling themselves. Aspartame may actually stimulate the appetite. And the food cravings evoked appear to be especially for fatty foods.

Caution: Honey is not recommended as a sugar alternative for children under 1 year old. It may contain bacteria which can cause infant botulism. If mold sensitive, use fresh fruits and fruit juices in place of commercially prepared fruits and juices.

❤ WHITE SUGAR

Substitutions:

1 cup sugar

> = 1 cup brown rice syrup powder
> = 1 cup *Fruitsource* sweetener, granulated or liquid
> = 3/4 cup maple syrup granules/syrup
> = 1/2 cup honey
> = 2 cups 100% barley malt (may contain corn)
> = 1 cup date sugar or pitted dates
> = 1 cup fruit juice sweetened spreadable fruit
> = 1 cup sun-ripened dried fruit, chopped, or soaked and puréed

= 1 cup *Sucanat* organic granulated
cane juice

Note: Decrease liquids in recipe by 25 percent when substituting liquids for dry ingredients.

❤ BROWN SUGAR

Substitutions:

1 cup brown sugar

= 1/2 or 3/4 cup maple mixture
(1 part maple syrup to 2 parts
maple syrup granules)
= 1 cup *Sucanat* organic granulated cane juice

❤ CONFECTIONER'S SUGAR

Substitutions:

1 cup confectioner's sugar

= 1 cup maple syrup gran-
ules powdered in
blender for 3 minutes,
or powdered by hand
using a rolling pin.
= 1 cup *Ohsawa* brown
rice syrup powder
= 1 cup date sugar (This
is merely ground dried

dates and makes a very satisfying white sugar alternative. Since it is not as fine as white sugar, I powder it in a blender when a recipe calls for powdered sugar.)

❤ MOLASSES

Use equal portions 100% brown rice syrup or *Fruitsource* liquid sweetener.

TAPIOCA STARCH

Substitutions:

1/2 tablespoon tapioca starch

= 1/2 tablespoon potato starch
= 21/2 teaspoons arrow-root starch
= 1 tablespoon flour (rice, rye, barley)
= 1 tablespoon corn starch

Do not use arrowroot starch in a recipe that has to be rewarmed as it loses its thickening capacity.

TEA, HOT OR ICED

Many herb teas are available that are caffeine free. However, if the concern is allergy and/or chemical contamination, the following suggestions are delicious and nutritious.

Substitutions:

1/2 teaspoon acerola cherry powder (contains approximately 85 mg vitamin C) dissolved in 1 cup hot (not boiling) water. Dash of lemon juice, optional. May be iced after dissolved.

Or 1/4 cup any juice + 3/4 cup boiling water.

VANILLA EXTRACT

If you want to eliminate the alcohol, sugar, and salt that most vanilla extracts contain, you can make your own.

Place a vanilla bean in a quart jar filled with flour or sugar. Leave in jar for at least 1 week before using. The longer the better. Use in place of separate vanilla and flour or vanilla and sugar.

1 teaspoon vanilla =

> **1 tsp.** *Cook's Vanilla Powder* (in a dextrose sugar base, but contains no alcohol), or
> 1/4 teaspoon ground vanilla bean

Bickford Laboratories makes a vanilla extract without alcohol, sugar or salt.

VINEGAR

Most commercial vinegars are manufactured from corn. They also contain yeast and yeast-like substances by the nature of their manufacture.

Cider vinegar is made from fermented apple juice.

Rice vinegar is made from fermented rice and is a low acid vinegar.

Substitution:

Fresh lemon juice may be used in recipes calling for vinegar. Use in equal proportions.

WHEAT BRAN

Substitutions:

In equal amounts:

> Oat bran
> Steel cut oats
> Rice bran
> Matzo meal, if wheat is not the problem

WHITE FLOUR

Substitutions:

> Spelt flour (a form of wheat)
> Whole wheat pastry flour
> Barley flour

Kamut flour (a form of wheat)
Oat flour

All are excellent. Use as you would white flour, in equal proportions.

Teff flour may also be used, but amounts are tricky. It is fine for crackers, pie crusts, and cookies.

Note: When substituting for white flour in cakes and muffins you will not get the same rise, so use carbonated spring water in place of liquid in recipes.

WHITE RICE

Substitutions:

In equal proportions:

> Brown rice
> Wild rice
> Millet
> Buckwheat groats (kasha)
> 100% quinoa
> Orzo pasta—very small durum wheat pasta that is shaped like rice and is the same size.

♥ KASHA PILAF (Roasted Buckwheat Kernels)

 1   cup kasha
 2   cups boiling water
 1   slightly beaten egg
 2   tablespoons high-oleic safflower oil
     Sea salt, to taste
 1   medium onion, sliced and sautéed
10   mushrooms, thin sliced and sautéed

Place kasha and beaten egg in saucepan, stirring to coat each kernel with egg. Place over medium heat stirring continuously with fork until all kernels are dry and separate. Remove pan from burner. Add boiling water, oil, onions and mushrooms, and cover. Return to burner and simmer for about 10 minutes, or until all water has been absorbed and kasha is tender. Serve plain or with brown gravy. If mold or yeast sensitive omit mushrooms. SERVES 4.

WINE

If you are asthmatic or allergic to sulfiting agents, you may wish to avoid drinking commercial wine. Sulfur dioxide, a sulfiting agent and post-harvest fumigant, is used on grapes as protection from bunch rot. There are approximately 80 other chemicals used in winemaking, but most of these additives and preservatives need not be listed on the label. Organic wines that are additive-free and preservative-free are available at health food stores; however, naturally fermented wines produce some sulfites as a natural by-product during fermentation.

Substitutions:

For cooking, use equal amounts of white grape juice or apple juice.

WINE MARINADE

- 1/4 cup vinegar
- 1/4 cup water
- 1 tablespoon *Fruitsource* liquid sweetener or organic brown rice syrup

Combine and use.

❤ WINE, SPARKLING

Substitutions:

For drinking, use equal parts carbonated spring water and one of the following:

> Cranberry/apple juice
> White grape juice
> Red grape juice
> Apple juice

YOGURT

Yogurt is a rich source of protein and contains essential vitamins and minerals. The protein in

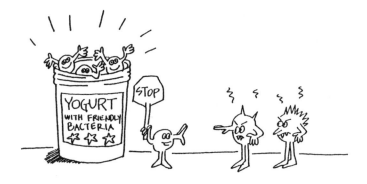

yogurt is more easily digested than the proteins in milk. The beneficial bacteria in yogurt work within the intestinal tract inhibiting the growth of unfriendly bacteria and facilitating the absorbtion of minerals and vitamins.

I prefer to make my own yogurt as it is simple, cost-effective, and free of sweetening agents, flavorings and other chemical additives. Check your health food store for fat-free, organic yogurt. The following recipes will enable you to make purer, fruited yogurt desserts that can be served as you would use any commercial sweetened yogurt.

Add 1 quart fat-free organic yogurt to any one of the following:

- 1/4 cup 100% maple syrup
- 4 tablespoons honey
- 6 tablespoons carob powder and honey, to taste

- 1 tablespoon *Cook's Vanilla Powder* alone, or in combination with 1/2 cup fruit juice sweetened spreadable fruit or for fruit-at-the-bottom style yogurt, simply add 2 tablespoons fresh fruit, at the bottom of an individual serving dish.

When cooking with yogurt, spare the heat. To keep the bacillus alive, keep the temperature below 120° F. Blend a little flour and water into the yogurt if you will be cooking it, in order to keep it from curdling. It is always best to stir the yogurt into the food after it has been removed from the heat.

Nondairy substitutions:

Tofu combined in a blender with sweetener of choice.

Several soy-based yogurts are available at health food stores. There are many fruit flavored styles available as well as vanilla flavored and plain.

Lowfat organic goat's milk or sheep's milk yogurt are also available at health food stores. *Yo-Goat*, a cultured goat's milk is also available.

SECTION THREE

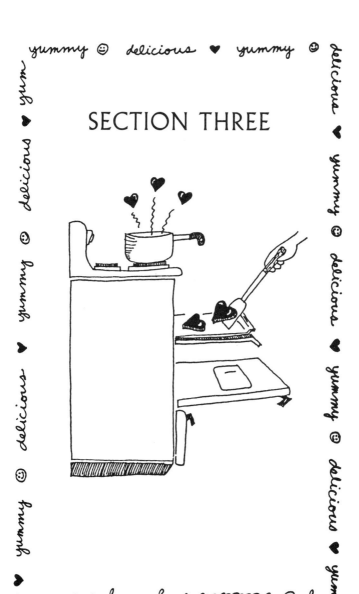

RECIPES

To make it easier for you to locate recipes which are free of dairy, wheat, gluten, eggs, and/or sugar, look for the symbols:

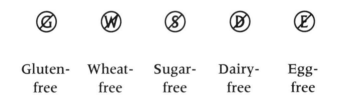

| Gluten-free | Wheat-free | Sugar-free | Dairy-free | Egg-free |

You will notice the absence of spices from most of my recipes. I use them only when absolutely necessary. A wonderful flavor and aroma result from just the right combinations of foods, without the addition of spices. We have been putting additional flavorings in our foods out of habit and because ''the recipe calls for it.'' For instance, salt, the most common offender, can be left out of any recipe. You may wish to continue salting at first, but when you feel brave, try using less and less each time, and you will be pleasantly surprised when your family stops asking you to "pass the salt shaker."

Be sure to check the Brand Name Product Guide to help you locate the specific allergen-free products I recommend.

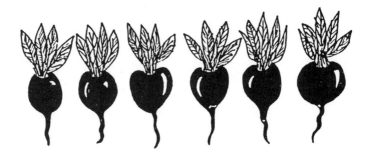

RECIPE INDEX

DIPS

♥ GARBANZO BEAN DIP

1 cup garbanzo beans, cooked and drained
(reserving 1 tablespoon liquid)
1 tablespoon extra virgin olive oil
1 teaspoon lemon juice
Bragg™ liquid aminos to taste
minced garlic to taste, optional
dash of paprika, optional

Purée beans in blender until smooth adding reserved liquid (only if needed) to blend. Add remaining ingredients and blend a few seconds. Chill. Serve heaped in a bowl as a dip for pieces of pita bread or romaine lettuce leaves. YIELD: 1 CUP.

♥ DILL WEED DIP

    2/3   cup *Walnut Acres No-Yolk Mayonnaise* (contains egg white)

    2/3   cup homemade fat-free yogurt cheese or kefir cheese (see page 45)

    1   green onion, minced

    1   tablespoon parsley, minced

    2   teaspoons dill weed, minced

    1   teaspoon sea salt

Mix together and serve with fresh vegetables for dipping. YIELD: APPROXIMATELY 1 1/2 CUPS.

CRACKERS & BREADS

♥ BARLEY BREAD STICKS

    2   cups barley flour

    1 1/2   tablespoons *Fruitsource Granulated Sweetener*

    3   tablespoons high-oleic safflower oil

    3/4   cup cold water

    1/4   teaspoon salt

    2   green onions, finely chopped, optional

Mix all ingredients well, except green onions, in bowl. Add green onions, and knead until mixed through. Tear off pieces and roll in palms into 1/2" thick strips. Place on greased cookie sheet and bake at 350° for 35 minutes, or until browned and firm to touch. YIELD: 4 SERVINGS.

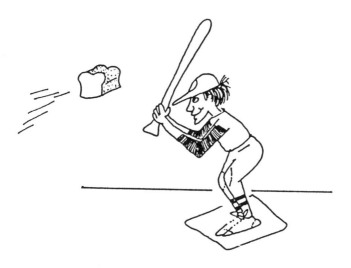

♥ SOUTHERN BATTER BREAD PUDDING

1   cup cornmeal
2   tablespoons non-aluminum baking powder
2   cups *Rice Dream Original Lite Rice Milk*
2   eggs (or substitutions, page 57)
1   cup boiling water
2   tablespoons 100% maple syrup
2   tablespoons melted ghee

In a large bowl, combine cornmeal and baking powder. Stir in milk. Then beat in eggs, add boiling water, maple syrup and ghee. Pour batter carefully into a greased 1 1/2 quart baking dish. Bake in pre-heated 375° oven for 35 minutes or until golden brown on top. Serve as a pudding or as an accompaniment to roast beef. SERVES 4 TO 6.

♥ ZUCCHINI BREAD

2	eggs + 1 egg white
1	cup extra virgin olive oil
4	ounces unsweetened pineapple juice
2	cups shredded zucchini
8	ounces fruit juice sweetened peach spreadable fruit preserves
3	cups rye flour
2	teaspoons baking soda
1/2	teaspoon non-aluminum baking powder (see page 33)
1	teaspoon cinnamon
1	teaspoon salt, optional
1	cup chopped walnuts
1	cup raisins

Beat eggs, add oil and pineapple juice and mix. Stir in zucchini and spreadable fruit. Combine dry ingredients and add to mixture. Add nuts and raisins. Bake in preheated 325° oven for one hour in greased loaf pan. YIELD: 2 LOAVES.

BEVERAGES

♥ APRICOT-MELON COOLER

1 cup cubed cantaloupe, chilled in freezer for an hour

1 cup unsweetened apricot nectar, chilled

1/2 cup soy apricot yogurt

honey to taste, optional

2 dashes of cinnamon, optional

Mix together in blender and serve immediately. SERVES 2.

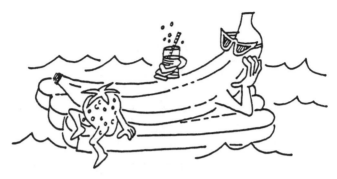

❤ BANANA-BERRY FLOAT

Ⓖ
Ⓦ
Ⓢ
Ⓓ
Ⓔ

2	medium-size bananas
6	large strawberries
1/2	cup strawberry soy yogurt
4	whole berries

Slice bananas and 6 strawberries and place in blender. Add 1/2 cup soy yogurt and blend. Add more soy yogurt to make 2 1/2 cups of mixture. Serve in tall glasses with 2 berries floating in each glass. Can be frozen into creamsicles (see page 00). SERVES: 2.

❤ CAROBANA SHAKE

Omit strawberries from above recipe and add 1 1/2 tablespoons carob and 2 teaspoons of brown rice syrup, or more, to taste.

❤ BROWN COW

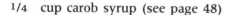

- 1/4 cup carob syrup (see page 48)
- 8   ounces carbonated spring water
- 2   scoops vanilla *Rice Dream Frozen Dessert*

Pour syrup in bottom of tall glass. Add about 1/2 cup of spring water. Stir to mix, and then add *Rice Dream.* Fill the glass with the rest of the spring water. SERVES 1.

❤ CAROB BANANA SHAKE

- 2   cups soy milk
- 1   tablespoon chopped dates
- 1/2 banana
- 1   teaspoon peanut butter
- 1   heaping tablespoon carob powder

Mix all ingredients in blender and serve. SERVES 2.

♥ CAROB TWO-WAY STRETCH

Ⓖ
Ⓦ
Ⓢ
Ⓓ
Ⓔ

    1   cup raw cashew nut milk (see page 76)
    1   cup *Rice Dream Original Lite rice milk*
   1/2 banana
    1   heaping teaspoon carob powder, or more, to taste

Mix all together in blender until smooth. May be served warm or cold for a nutritious breakfast drink. (If using nut milk stir constantly while warming on low heat, as nut milk thickens and becomes a pudding quickly. If too late, serve as a pudding!) Serve immediately! Do not refrigerate. SERVES 1 AS A DRINK OR 2 AS A PUDDING.

♥ CRANBERRY FIZZ

Ⓖ
Ⓦ
Ⓢ
Ⓓ
Ⓔ

   1/4 cup unsweetened cranberry nectar, chilled
   3/4 cup sparkling spring water, chilled
    1   tablespoon *Fruitsource Liquid Sweetener*

Mix and serve. SERVES 1.

♥ DOUBLE DATE-NUT SHAKE

1 1/2 cups almond nut milk (see page 76)
1/2   cup pitted dates, chopped
1/4   cup toasted pecans, finely chopped
1   cup frozen vanilla soy yogurt
1/8   teaspoon cinnamon
1/8   teaspoon vanilla, optional

Mix all together in blender and serve immediately.
SERVES 3.

♥ CREAM OF THE CROP COOLER

1/3   cup *Horizon* organic fat-free yogurt
2/3   cup beet juice, chilled
1/4   cup shredded beets
1   teaspoon *Fruitsource Liquid Sweetener* to taste,
         optional

Blend plain yogurt with beet juice and sweetener
in blender until smooth. Add shredded beets. Serve
chilled. SERVES 1.

♥ ISLANDER SMOOTHY

  1/2 cup papaya juice
  1/2 cup organic fat-free yogurt
  1 small banana, mashed
  1 tablespoon coconut, finely grated

Whip all in blender until smooth. SERVES 1.

♥ TOMATO VIT "A" JUICE SUPREME

  1 quart homemade stewed tomatoes
  1 cut-up green pepper
    a handful of washed and drained parsley

Press stewed tomatoes through a sieve to remove seeds and skins. Pour juice into a saucepan with green pepper and parsley and simmer about one-half hour. Strain. Refrigerate before serving. YIELD: APPROXIMATELY 1 QUART.

SALADS

♥ POTATO SALAD I

3	medium potatoes, cooked and cubed
2	celery stalks, chopped
1	green onion with top, chopped
1	small green pepper, chopped
2	hard-cooked egg whites, chopped
1/2	cup mayo-delicious (see page 68) or other yolk-free mayonnaise mixed with equal parts organic fat-free yogurt.

Mix all ingredients together and chill. SERVES 4.

♥ POTATO SALAD II

4	medium potatoes, cooked and cubed
2	celery stalks, chopped
1	green onion with top, chopped
1	green pepper, chopped
1	red pepper, chopped
2/3	cup vanilla soy yogurt
2	tablespoons *Ohsawa Brown Rice Syrup Powder* dry mustard, to taste

Mix all ingredients together and chill. SERVES 4.

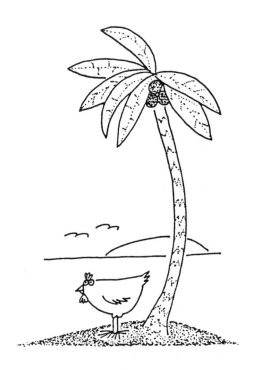

♥ ISLANDER CHICKEN SALAD

ⓖ ⓦ ⓢ ⓓ

1	cooked chicken breast, cubed
1/2	cup celery, sliced
2	green onions with tops, sliced
1	cup fresh pineapple, cubed
1	cup seedless green grapes
	few sprigs of parsley

Pineapple-Coconut Dressing (see page 124)

Toss all together, garnishing the top with parsley sprigs. SERVES 4.

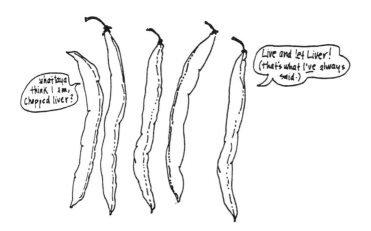

♥ PSEUDO CHOPPED LIVER

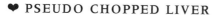

2	eggs, hard cooked (whites only if you prefer)
1	large onion, chopped fine and sautéed in oil
1	package frozen or fresh green beans, steamed until crisp-tender and well drained
1/4	cup walnuts
	sea salt and pepper, to taste

Place all ingredients except seasonings in food processor and blend, using off-on switch until almost smooth. Add seasoning.

Serve on crackers as an appetizer, or as a salad garnished with sliced fresh vegetables. Makes a delicious sandwich. YIELD: APPROXIMATELY 1 1/2 CUP.

SALAD DRESSINGS

♥ CREAMY SALAD DRESSING

2	hard-cooked eggs
6	tablespoons plain soy yogurt
4	teaspoons extra virgin olive oil
1	green onion, diced
	sea salt, to taste
1/4	teaspoon lemon juice, optional

Put all ingredients in blender and blend for 1 minute until smooth. If made the day before, mix in blender again before serving.

YIELD: APPROXIMATELY 1/2 CUP.

♥ PINEAPPLE-COCONUT DRESSING

1/4	cup shredded coconut, toasted
1/4	cup slivered almonds, toasted
3/4	cup plain soy yogurt
3	tablespoons *Walnut Acres* No-Yolk mayonnaise (contains egg white)
4	tablespoons pineapple juice
1	tablespoon fruit juice sweetened orange marmalade

Mix together well, and chill. Delicious as a topping over fruit salad. YIELD: 1 CUP.

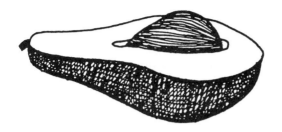

♥ GREEN GODDESS SALAD DRESSING

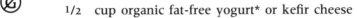

- 1/2 cup organic fat-free yogurt* or kefir cheese
- 1/2 large avocado
- 1 green onion, chopped
- 1/2 cup extra virgin olive oil
- 1 tablespoon water
- 1/2 teaspoon lemon juice
  sea salt, to taste
  garlic, minced, optional

Put all ingredients in blender until smooth. If using plain yogurt in place of Kefir cheese, omit water.
YIELD: 1 CUP.

*For dairy-free version use lemon soy yogurt.

❤ FRENCH STYLE DRESSING

3	tablespoons *Fruitsource Liquid Sweetener*
2	teaspoons apple cider vinegar
6	tablespoons extra virgin olive oil
1	medium onion, chopped
1	garlic clove, minced
1	very large tomato, blanched and peeled

Combine the first five ingredients until well-processed. Add tomato and process until the tomato is in tiny pieces. Refrigerate until needed. Shake well before using.

YIELD: APPROXIMATELY 1 CUP.

SOUPS

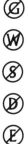

♥ CREAM OF POTATO SOUP

4	medium potatoes, cut in bite-size pieces
	spring water to just cover potatoes in 4 1/2 quart pot
2	tablespoons extra virgin olive oil, optional
2	green onions with tops, sliced
	sea salt, or *Bragg Liquid Aminos* to taste
2	stalks celery, sliced diagonally and steamed until tender, optional

Cook potatoes in covered pot, until just done. Remove 1/2 cup of cooked potatoes, with a little broth, and place in blender, mixing until smooth and pasty. Return potato paste to pot, using a spatula for easy removal. Stir until potato paste and broth are smooth, being careful not to mash the remaining potato chunks. Add olive oil, onion and steamed celery, and simmer for 5 minutes before serving. YIELD: 4 CUPS.

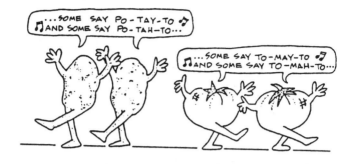

♥ POTATO SOUP SUPREME

4	medium potatoes, peeled and cubed
2 1/2	cups water
2	large carrots, sliced
2	tablespoons extra virgin olive oil, optional
1	handful fresh parsley sprigs
	sea salt, or *Bragg Liquid Aminos*, to taste

Cook potatoes in enough water to cover till tender but not mushy, and set aside. Steam carrots until very tender. Place carrots, oil and 1/2 cup of cubed potatoes in food processor and blend until smooth. Mixture will be thick. Fold mixture into remaining potatoes and potato water in pot. Stir gently until liquids are blended, being careful not to mash remaining potato cubes. Add sea salt and parsley.
YIELD: 4 TO 5 SERVINGS.

Note: Thin with water reserved from carrots to desired consistency.

♥ CABBAGE POTATO SOUP

1	medium onion, chopped
1	half head of cabbage, shredded
2	tablespoons extra virgin olive oil
3	scrubbed, unpeeled baking potatoes in bite size cubes
	sea salt or *Bragg Liquid Aminos*

Sauté onion and cabbage in olive oil and set aside. Cook cubed potatoes until fork tender in enough water to cover. Do not overcook. Scoop out 1/2 cup potatoes with slotted spoon and purée in blender. Then add back to the soup. Stir to thicken until the broth is smooth. Add sautéed vegetables, including remaining oil in pan. Simmer 30 minutes. Soup will continue to thicken as it simmers. SERVES 4.

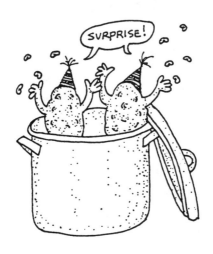

❤ POTATO BEAN SOUP SURPRISE

2	potatoes, cubed
2	carrots, cubed
8	ounces organic diced tomatoes
1	115 ounce can organic black beans, with broth
1/3	cup reserved potato water
31/2	ounces whole cranberry sauce
1	tablespoon minced onion
3	tablespoons *Fruitsource Granulated Sweetener*
	sea salt, or miso to taste

Steam potatoes and carrots in water until tender and set aside. Place the remaining ingredients in a large pot. Add steamed carrots and potatoes, setting aside the remaining water. Simmer 1/2 hour. Add remaining water to desired consistency, if needed, as soup tends to thicken as it simmers. SERVES 6.

❤ INSTANT CREAM OF TOMATO SOUP

Ⓖ Ⓦ Ⓢ Ⓓ Ⓔ

| 2 | cups organic tomato juice, heated |
| 2 | tablespoons plain soy yogurt, slightly warmed |

Add small amount of heated juice to soy yogurt in blender and blend. Slowly add the rest of the juice and whir a few seconds. Serve immediately, or put back on stove until warm enough to serve. SERVES 2.

❤ TOMATO BISQUE

Ⓖ Ⓦ Ⓢ Ⓓ Ⓔ

3	cups of cold Hi-C tomato soup (see page 132)
16	ounces tofu, well-drained and chopped
2	green onions, tops only, chopped

Blend soup and tofu together in food processor until smooth. Place in saucepan and cook over medium heat until hot. Do not boil. Garnish with green onion tops. SERVES 4.

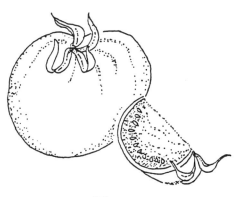

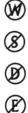

♥ COLD ORGANIC HI-C TOMATO
SOUP/JUICE

In food processor, combine the following organic ingredients:

1	16 ounce can organic diced tomatoes
1/2	cucumber, peeled and chopped
1	small green pepper, chopped
1	small carrot, grated
	powder from 2-1000 mg vitamin C (citric acid) capsules
4–5	sprigs of fresh dill
1/3	teaspoon sea salt

Blend on high until smooth. Serve cold in soup plates.

Garnish with a dollop of soy yogurt and chopped green onion tops. Make early in the day so that flavors have a chance to blend. When served as juice, may be served with a celery stalk for garnish. SERVES 4.

❤ QUICK CREAM OF CORN SYRUP

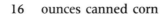

16	ounces canned corn
1	cup *Rice Dream Original Lite Rice Milk*
2	tablespoons organic ghee
1	tablespoon *Fruitsource Granular Sweetener*
	sea salt and pepper to taste
2	tablespoons of brown rice syrup

Pour contents of can, including liquid, into food processor or blender long enough to mash corn. Some chunks will remain. Pour into saucepan. Add remaining ingredients. Cook over medium heat stirring constantly to prevent burning. When soup starts to boil, remove from heat and serve immediately. MAKES 2 LARGE SERVINGS.

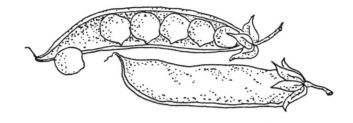

♥ FRESH CREAM OF PEA SOUP

2	packages frozen peas (12.3 ounce size)
1	carrot, chopped fine
1/2	cup *Rice Dream Original Lite Rice Milk*
	parsley for garnish

Steam carrots and peas until tender. Remove peas and place in blender. Purée with 8 tablespoons reserved cooking water. Some pieces will remain. Return to cooking pot, and add carrots and rice milk. Cook on medium heat stirring constantly just until mixture boils. Garnish with sprigs of parsley. SERVES 4.

MAIN DISHES

♥ CHINESE EGG ROLLS

PASTRY:

3	eggs, beaten
3/4	cup water
1/2	teaspoon salt
3/4	cup whole wheat pastry flour
1	tablespoon high-oleic safflower oil

Beat all ingredients together, except oil. In a 7" skillet, heat oil and pour in a scant 1/3 cup of batter to make a thin pancake. Brown on one side only. Repeat process until all batter is used.

FILLING:

1	cup chopped celery
1/2	cup chopped green onions with tops
1 1/2	cups red cabbage, shredded
1	cup cooked chicken, cubed
2	tablespoons high-oleic safflower oil
1/2	cup alfalfa sprouts
1	egg white, beaten
	salt and pepper, optional

Sauté celery, onions, and cabbage in oil for 5 minutes. Add chicken and sprouts and cool mixture about 15 minutes. Place 1 heaping tablespoon of filling at one end, uncooked side, of each pancake and roll up, tucking ends in as you go. Seal with egg white and refrigerate for several hours. Fry in oil until brown. Serve with Chinese Hot Sauce (see page 84). YIELD: 6 ROLLS.

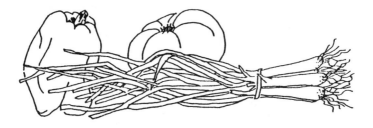

♥ BROWN RICE AND VEGETABLE SAUTÉ

Ⓖ
Ⓦ
Ⓢ
Ⓓ
Ⓔ

1	large onion, cut in 8 wedges and separated
2	green peppers, sliced in medium size pieces
2	tomatoes, each cut in 8 wedges
2	cups brown rice, cooked
	sea salt, to taste
	extra virgin olive oil, as needed

In an electric skillet on medium heat, sauté onion and green peppers until almost browned. Add tomatoes, stirring constantly, until just heated through, being careful not to boil away liquids. Season to taste. Divide into two portions and pour over heated brown rice. SERVES 2.

❤ STIR-FRY CHINESE RICE

2	small green onions with tops, chopped
1	egg + 2 whites, beaten
2	cups brown rice, cooked and warmed
1	cup chicken, cooked and cubed, optional
3	tablespoons defatted chicken stock or water (to defat, see page 35)
	sea salt, to taste
	sesame oil for frying
2	tablespoons unsalted, dry roasted cashew nuts, chopped

Sauté onions in oil for a few minutes and pour in beaten eggs. Scramble mixture into small pieces by constantly stirring with a fork. Lower heat to simmer and add rice, chicken, chicken stock and salt. Stir to mix and cover for a few more minutes to heat thoroughly, adding more oil if necessary. Garnish with cashew nuts. SERVES 2 OR 3.

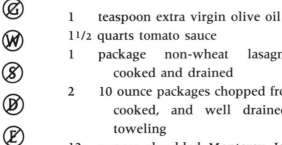

♥ SPINACH LASAGNA

1   teaspoon extra virgin olive oil
1 1/2 quarts tomato sauce
1   package non-wheat lasagna noodles,
     cooked and drained
2   10 ounce packages chopped frozen spinach,
     cooked, and well drained on paper
     toweling
12   ounces shredded Monterey Jack style soy
     cheese
3   tablespoons grated Romano style soy cheese
     sea salt, optional
     minced garlic, optional

Oil an 8 1/2" × 12" baking pan and place a small
amount of sauce over it to moisten. Lay down a
single layer of noodles. Spread half of the spinach
over the noodles, followed by half of the Monterey
Jack grated soy cheese. Top with about one-third
of the remaining sauce and repeat these layers
once, ending with noodles. Place the remaining
sauce over noodles to just cover and sprinkle with
grated Romano soy cheese. Bake uncovered in preheated 350° oven for 45 minutes. May be prepared
early in day and refrigerated, taking out one-half
hour before cooking. SERVES 6.

♥ SPINACH FRITTATA

1/2	package frozen chopped spinach
6	egg whites, beaten medium stiff
1/2	small onion, chopped and sautéed
	extra virgin olive oil for frying

Steam spinach, drain well and press between two layers of paper toweling to remove excess moisture. Pour beaten egg whites into greased electric skillet on medium heat. Spread spinach and sautéed onions evenly over top of egg whites. When pancake is brown underneath, flip over and brown lightly. The secret to frying egg whites successfully is to maintain a medium heat and use a well-oiled skillet. SERVES 2.

♥ VEGETABLE SPAGHETTI SAUCE

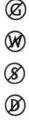

8	ounces tomato paste
1	16 ounce can diced tomatoes with liquid
6	tablespoons unsweetened peach spreadable fruit preserves
2	carrots, diagonally sliced
1	small onion, chopped
2	green peppers, cut in chunks
2	medium zucchini, cut in chunks
1	clove garlic, minced
2	tablespoons extra virgin olive oil
	sea salt or *Bragg Liquid Aminos* to taste

Combine tomato paste and diced tomatoes with spreadable fruit preserves and add water, if needed, to consistency you desire. Mix well and bring back to a quick boil. Turn to simmer and prepare vegetables. Steam carrots until al dente (slightly undercooked). Sauté onions, peppers, zucchini, and minced garlic in olive oil until vegetables are limp. Add to tomato mixture along with carrots. Continue simmering for 30 minutes. Add sea salt or liquid aminos to taste.

YIELD: APPROXIMATELY 1 PINT.

♥ QUICK BLINTZES

8	slices spelt* bread
16	ounces tofu, drained and crumbled
1	egg + 2 whites, well beaten and set aside
1/2	cup raisins, softened in water and drained
1/4	teaspoon non-irradiated cinnamon
1	tablespoon *Ohsawa Brown Rice Syrup Powder*, or more to taste
	oil as needed, to pan-fry

Cut off and discard crusts from bread. With rolling pin, flatten bread to about 1/8" thick, without tearing. Mix tofu, raisins, cinnamon, rice syrup powder, and 1 teaspoon of beaten egg together for filling. Place 1 tablespoon of filling on edge of flattened piece of bread and roll jelly-roll fashion, keeping filling inside as you go. Hold securely as you roll each blintz through the remaining beaten eggs and place in electric skillet on medium heat, turning to brown on all sides. Place a dollop of soy yogurt on each blintz at serving time. SERVES 2.

*Spelt is a type of wheat that many wheat-sensitive individuals can tolerate.

♥ VEGGIE SANDWICH

 2   slices 100% rye bread (slightly warmed to
      soften)
      sliced tomato
      chopped green onion
      alfalfa sprouts

Heap slices of tomato, green onion and alfalfa sprouts on the bread. Top with second slice, and enjoy.

♥ MONTE CRISTO SANDWICH BAKE

12   slices 100% rye bread
12   1 ounce slices Swiss style soy cheese
 2   eggs + 3 egg whites
 2   cups *Rice Dream Original Lite Rice Milk*
 1   teaspoon sea salt
      organic sauerkraut

Using a 9" × 13" greased pan, arrange 6 slices of bread to cover bottom. Place 1 slice of soy cheese on each piece of bread and cover with 6 remaining bread slices, forming 6 sandwiches. Beat eggs, rice milk and salt together well and pour over sandwiches. Place in refrigerator about 4 hours or overnight. Bake in preheated 350° oven for approximately 35 minutes until browned and firm and sandwiches can be separated easily with a knife. Place a dollop of warmed sauerkraut on top of each sandwich. SERVES: 6.

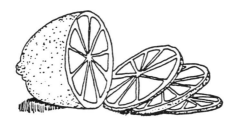

♥ LEMON CHICKEN

2   chicken breasts, split, skinned and boned
3   tablespoons extra virgin olive oil
1/2 lemon
1   handful fresh parsley sprigs
     sea salt

Sauté chicken breasts in olive oil on medium-high heat till lightly browned on each side. Cook 3–5 minutes longer on each side at a reduced temperature until chicken is fork tender. Remove chicken to serving dish and set aside. Squeeze lemon into pan. Add parsley, sea salt, and stir to combine juices, then pour over chicken and serve immediately. SERVES 4.

Note: For Chicken Tarragon, sauté fresh chopped tarragon and chopped green onions in the olive oil in place of lemon juice and parsley.

♥ SESAME CHICKEN WITH PEAPODS

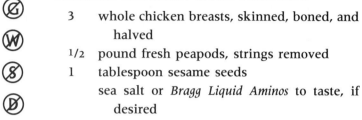

3   whole chicken breasts, skinned, boned, and
    halved
1/2 pound fresh peapods, strings removed
1   tablespoon sesame seeds
    sea salt or *Bragg Liquid Aminos* to taste, if
    desired

Place chicken pieces in enough water to cover and bring to a boil over high heat. Reduce heat to medium-low. Cover and poach for a half hour or until fork tender. While chicken is poaching, steam peapods until *al denté* and prepare pineapple-orange sauce below.

PINEAPPLE-ORANGE SAUCE

1 1/2 cups unsweetened pineapple juice
1/2 cup unsweetened orange marmalade
3   tablespoons arrowroot starch
    a few drops of *Bragg Liquid Aminos*

Combine pineapple juice with orange marmalade. Cook and stir in sauce pan on medium-low until thoroughly blended. Remove 1/2 cup of the mixture and stir in arrowroot starch until well blended, then return to saucepan and continue cooking until mixture thickens and is clear. Add liquid aminos. Turn heat to low and simmer an additional 5 minutes.

Arrange chicken breasts on a platter. Serve with peapods and spoon pineapple orange sauce over chicken. Garnish with sesame seeds. SERVES 6.

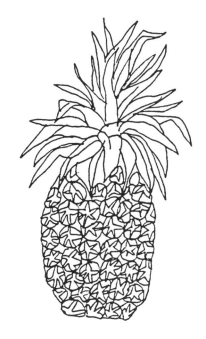

❤ PINEAPPLE-ALMOND CHICKEN

2   whole chicken breasts, split, skinned and
        boned
2   tablespoons extra virgin olive oil
1/2 small head of cabbage, coarsely shredded
6   ounces unsweetened pineapple juice
1   tablespoon cornstarch
1   10 ounce package frozen peas, steamed
1   6 ounce package slivered almonds
     Bragg Liquid Aminos, to taste, if desired
1   8 ounce package 100% buckwheat noodles
        (soba)

Slice chicken crosswise into strips. Sauté in olive oil over medium heat until lightly browned on both sides. Push chicken to the side of the pan and add cabbage. Sauté cabbage, stirring until limp (just a few minutes). You may have to add about 2 ounces of water to keep cabbage from sticking. Mix cabbage and chicken together, and continue cooking until chicken is fork tender. Turn off heat and set aside. Mix cornstarch with three table-spoons of the pineapple juice until blended, then add remaining juice and stir together. Blend sauce with chicken mixture in pan and cook until thick-ened. Add steamed peas. Prepare noodles as pack-age directs. Serve chicken mixture over cooked noodles and sprinkle with almonds. SERVES 4.

❤ GEFILTE CHICKEN

2   skinless and boneless chicken breasts (about 1 pound)

1/4   cup *Rice Dream Original Lite Rice Milk*

2   tablespoons oat flour

1   egg, beaten

1   small carrot, finely grated

1   small onion, chopped fine

1   tablespoon dill

1/2   teaspoon sea salt or liquid aminos to taste

1   tablespoon extra virgin olive oil

Poach chicken breasts in enough water to cover until fork tender. Chill and remove the congealed fat. Place chicken in food processor and process until it resembles flakes. Remove to a bowl and mix with remaining ingredients except olive oil. Grease the bottom and the sides of six muffin wells. Spoon chicken mixture into muffin wells pressing firmly. Bake at 350° in preheated oven for 45 minutes or until edges turn brown. Remove from oven. Use a knife to loosen edges before removing from wells. SERVES 6.

Note: This recipe has been adapted from a traditional Jewish baked fish recipe. It may be served hot or cold.

♥ TURKEY SCALLOPINI

1/2	turkey breast, skinned and boned
1	cup oat flour
3	tablespoons extra virgin olive oil
3/4	cup unsweetened white grape juice
2	tablespoons oat flour for thickening gravy
	sea salt and pepper to taste

Slice turkey breast crosswise into half inch cutlets. Pound to flatten slightly and set aside. Pour flour into bowl and set aside. Heat 3 tablespoons olive oil in frying pan on medium heat. Rinse turkey cutlets under running water, dredge with flour, and carefully place cutlets in heated frying pan. Sauté until nicely browned on each side. Remove from pan and reduce heat to simmer. Combine 2 tablespoons of oat flour with 1/4 cup of grape juice, mix well and add to remaining grape juice. Pour into pan while stirring and scraping the bottom of pan to combine juices. Add salt and pepper to taste. Stir until gravy is smooth and thick. Pour over cutlets and serve. SERVES 4.

♥ TURKEY ROLL UP

13/4 lb. ground turkey breast
2   egg whites
1/2   cup *Rice Dream Original Lite Rice Milk*
1/2   cup crushed whole wheat cracker crumbs
      (or any tolerated crumbs)
      extra virgin olive oil
1   cup chopped onions
1/4   cup chopped parsley
1/2   cup apricot unsweetened spreadable fruit
      sea salt or *Bragg Liquid Aminos* to taste

Blend turkey with egg whites and rice milk. Set aside. Lightly grease a 15 inch long piece of 100% unbleached baking paper. Spread the turkey mixture onto it by shaping it into an 8 × 10 inch rectangle. Set aside.

Sauté onions and combine with crushed cracker crumbs and parsley and spread evenly on top of turkey mixture. Season with sea salt or sprinkle with liquid aminos. Roll up firmly, jelly roll fashion, by lifting the paper to form a loaf. Begin rolling with the smaller edge, and discard paper when finished. Roll off of the paper onto a lightly greased baking dish. Place in a preheated 350° oven for 30 minutes. Spoon fruit spread evenly over the top. Return to oven and bake until done (approximately 15 minutes). SERVES 6.

❤ TURKEY JOES

2	lbs. ground turkey breast
2	tablespoons extra virgin olive oil
14	ounces of tomato purée
1/2	cup of water (approximately)
4	tablespoons maple syrup granules
1/2	cup whole cranberry sauce
	sea salt or *Bragg Liquid Aminos* to taste

Sauté ground turkey in the olive oil until the meat turns white. Add remaining ingredients and cook on low, stirring occasionally for 15 minutes. Serve Turkey Joes piled high on gluten-free hamburger buns spread with egg-free honey mustard.

Note: Add a little extra tomato purée and you have a delicious spaghetti sauce.

❤ MATZOH BREI (Pancake)

2   sheets of whole wheat matzoh
     hot water
2   eggs + 4 egg whites, beaten
     pinch of salt
2   tablespoons high-oleic safflower oil

Break matzoh into bite-size pieces and place in bowl of hot water to soften for a few minutes. Remove and drain well. Squeeze out the moisture. Combine softened matzoh in bowl with eggs and salt. Heat oil in electric skillet and pour in matzoh mix. It should cover bottom of pan, forming one large pancake. When browned on bottom, cut in half to flip (unless you are an expert flipper) to brown other side. Serve with brown rice syrup or apple sauce.

For *vegetable* matzoh brei, fold in 2 cups fresh steamed spinach and 3/4 cups strained diced organic tomatoes into matzoh-egg mixture before sautéing. Eliminate above topping. SERVES 2.

♥ FARMER'S CHOP SUEY

(G) (W) (S) (E)

12	ounces low-fat cottage cheese
1/4	cup organic fat-free yogurt
1	tomato, diced
1	green pepper, diced
1	green onion, diced
1	small carrot, sliced thin
2	radishes, sliced thin
	a handful of sprouts

Mix cheese and yogurt together in a large bowl. Mix in vegetables. May be served warm, if desired.
SERVES TWO HUNGRY PEOPLE.

♥ RICE À LA RED CABBAGE CASSEROLE

(G) (W) (S) (D) (E)

1/2	head red cabbage, medium size, sliced in 1/2" strips
1	large red apple, peeled and cored
1 1/2	cups brown rice, cooked and drained
1	medium size onion, chopped, optional
3	tablespoons high-oleic safflower oil
	sea salt, optional

Sauté onion and cabbage in large electric skillet until golden. Slice apples into bite size pieces and add to cabbage, cooking until slightly brown. Add cooked rice and sauté until heated through.
SERVES 2.

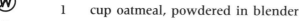 NUT BURGERS SUPREME

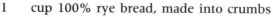

1	cup oatmeal, powdered in blender
1	cup 100% rye bread, made into crumbs
1	cup walnuts, finely chopped
1	onion, chopped and sautéed in oil
3	tablespoons apple butter
2	tablespoons high-oleic safflower oil

Mix all ingredients together, except oil, adding just enough hot water to form into patties. After shaping into four patties, refrigerate for at least an hour. Brown on both sides in oiled skillet.

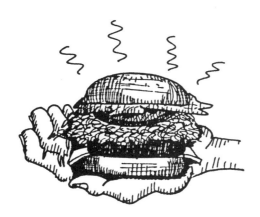

❤ QUINOA AND BEAN CASSEROLE

Ⓖ Ⓦ Ⓢ Ⓓ Ⓔ

1	cup quinoa
1	16 ounce can tomatoes, diced
1	cup celery, chopped
1	small onion, chopped
1	cup green pepper, chopped
1	tablespoon extra virgin olive oil
1	16 ounce can kidney beans, well drained and rinsed
1	teaspoon sea salt

Prepare quinoa as package directs and add tomatoes. Set aside. Sauté vegetables, with the exception of the beans, in olive oil. Add quinoa mixture, kidney beans and sea salt. Mix well. Grease the bottom and sides of a one quart casserole. Turn quinoa mixture into casserole and bake in a preheated 350° oven for approximately 30–45 minutes. SERVES 6.

❤ NUT LOAF/STUFFING

1	cup 100% rye bread made into crumbs (dried)
1	cup chopped celery
1	cup chopped pecans
2	tablespoons chopped parsley
2	tablespoons diced onion
1	egg + 2 egg whites, beaten
1	cup organic fat-free yogurt
2	tablespoons organic ghee
	sea salt, optional

Two hours before serving, mix ingredients together and spoon into a greased loaf pan. Let stand 45 minutes, then bake in preheated 350° oven for 50 minutes. May be served as a main dish with gravy, or used as a stuffing. YIELD: 1 LOAF.

♥ IRISH POTATO PANCAKES

Whir in blender:

- 1 egg
- 3 green onions, chopped
- 2 tablespoons matzo meal
- 1/2 teaspoon sea salt

Add:

- 3 potatoes, peeled and cubed

Mix until almost smooth. Mixture will be light green due to the green onion. Heat about one-half inch of high-oleic safflower oil in electric skillet. Drop scant 1/2 cupfuls potato mixture into hot oil. Cook until brown and crisp on bottom. Turn once to brown on other side. Then remove to drain on paper toweling. Can be kept warm in 200° oven until all are done. Serve with unsweetened applesauce and soy yogurt. YIELD: 8 TO 10.

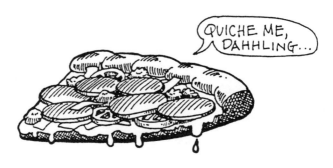

QUICHE ME, DAHHLING...

♥ PIZZA QUICHE

CRUST:

2	cups barley flour or kamut* flour
1/2	teaspoon sea salt
1/2	cup high-oleic safflower oil
1/4	cup water

Grease a 14 inch pizza pan and set aside. Mix flour with salt. Add oil and water and mix all together. Form into a ball. Place dough between two pieces of waxed paper and roll into a circle about 1/8" thick. Place dough on pan and flute edge. Using a pastry brush, spread the crust with about 1 teaspoon of oil.

Then place on crust, in order:

2	cups tomato sauce
3/4	cup chopped bell peppers, sautéed
3/4	cup chopped green onions, sautéed
5	ounces chopped, frozen spinach, drained very well
7	ounces shredded Monterey Jack style soy cheese

Sprinkle grated Romano style soy cheese lightly over all. Bake in preheated 450° oven for 15 to 20 minutes, until crust is browned on edges. Crust will be flaky. SERVES 2.

*Kamut flour is a type of wheat that many wheat-sensitive persons can tolerate. For gluten-free version use teff flour.

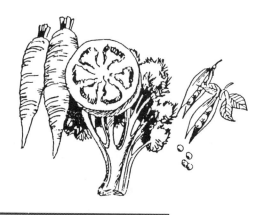

VEGETABLE SIDE DISHES

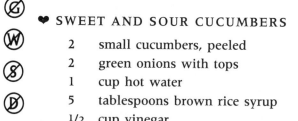

♥ SWEET AND SOUR CUCUMBERS

2	small cucumbers, peeled
2	green onions with tops
1	cup hot water
5	tablespoons brown rice syrup
1/2	cup vinegar

Slice cucumbers crosswise in paper-thin slices and place in a pint jar. Slice green onions once lengthwise and then crosswise into small pieces and add to cucumbers. Set aside. In a small bowl combine hot water and syrup, stirring until dissolved; then add vinegar. Pour vinegar mixture over onions and cucumbers in jar, stir to mix, cover and place in refrigerator at least one day before serving. The longer it cures, the tastier it becomes. SERVES 6 TO 8.

♥ TOMATO PUDDING

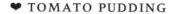

1 1/2 cups tomato sauce
3 tablespoons brown rice syrup
1 1/2 teaspoons lemon juice
2 tablespoons organic ghee, melted
5 pieces of 100% rye bread, toasted

Blend tomato sauce with rice syrup, lemon juice and ghee and place in a 1 1/2 quart casserole with cover. Break toast into large bite-size pieces and mix into sauce so that each piece is moistened. Bake in preheated 350° oven, covered, for 20 minutes. Remove cover and bake until browned and slightly crusted on top (about 10 to 15 minutes longer). SERVES 4.

♥ THE CARROT MASH

6 medium carrots, sliced and steamed
2 tablespoons organic ghee
salt to taste, optional

Place carrots in food processor and purée, adding ghee through feed tube. Serve like mashed potatoes. SERVES 4.

❤ SWEET POTATO PANCAKES

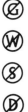

2	large sweet potatoes
3	egg whites
4	tablespoons potato flour
1/2	teaspoon sea salt
2	tablespoons extra virgin olive oil

Peel and grate sweet potatoes. Place potatoes in blender or food processor. Add remaining ingredients except olive oil and process. Mixture should be quite lumpy in texture. Do not overblend. If batter becomes overblended, add more flour as needed, to prevent pancakes from losing their shape. Generously grease a sheet cake pan with olive oil. Drop batter on cookie sheet—approximately 3 tablespoons per pancake. Flatten slightly. Bake in preheated 350° oven for approximately 20 minutes on each side. Turn gently with spatula when lightly browned on one side. Pancakes may have a tendency to crumble. Serve with unsweetened applesauce.

SERVES 2 AS A MAIN DISH. SERVES 4 AS A SIDE DISH.

SAUCES

♥ NO-COOK CATSUP

6	ounces tomato paste
3	tablespoons lemon juice
1/4	teaspoon allspice
1/4	teaspoon cinnamon
	Fruitsource Liquid Sweetener, to taste
	minced onion, optional

Place all ingredients in blender until smooth. Mix in water, 2 tablespoons at a time, until desired thickness. Refrigerate in covered jar. Use in 2 weeks. YIELD: 3/4 CUP.

♥ MAGICAL HOLLANDAISE SAUCE

3	tablespoons organic ghee
2	tablespoons teff flour
1	egg yolk
1	cup organic fat-free yogurt
1/2	teaspoon lemon juice, optional
1/4	teaspoon sea salt, optional

In top of double boiler melt ghee, add flour and stir to blend. Cool slightly and whisk in egg yolk. Add yogurt slowly and return to medium heat, stirring constantly, until thickened. Add lemon juice and sea salt. YIELD: APPROXIMATELY 1 CUP.

♥ GREEK YOGURT-CUCUMBER SAUCE

Ⓖ
Ⓦ
Ⓢ
Ⓔ

1	cup low-fat goat's milk yogurt
1	cucumber, peeled, seeded and sliced paper thin
1	teaspoon lemon juice
1	green onion with tops, finely chopped
1	tablespoon chopped parsley
1	garlic clove, minced, optional
	sea salt, to taste

Combine all ingredients and place in refrigerator in a covered container the night before serving. Serve as a side dish or mixed with chopped raw vegetables and placed in pita pockets.

MISCELLANEOUS

♥ PURE AND SIMPLE BUTTER

1   pint organic whipping cream

Pour whipping cream into deep bowl, and using electric beaters, whip until butter and milk separate (about 10 minutes). Pour off milk and save to drink. Press remaining milk out of butter with a spatula and drain. Place butter in a covered glass dish and refrigerate. Keeps about 1 week in the summer and 2 weeks in the winter. You may freeze it to store for longer periods.

This is especially nice if you have a pesticide-free local source for cream. If not, you can still eliminate the extra processing required to make butter and also eliminate the coloring used in making commercial butter. It will have a natural yellow color to it anyway. YIELD: APPROXIMATELY 1 1/4 CUPS.

♥ MY EGG-FREE MAYO

2   tablespoons brown rice syrup
8   ounces Kefir cheese
1/2 teaspoon dark mustard
     sea salt, to taste
     lemon juice, to taste, optional

Mix all ingredients together for a thick and delicious salad dressing that will fool any mayoholic!

DESSERTS

💜 FORGOTTEN MERINGUES

3	egg whites
1	cup *Ohsawa Brown Rice Syrup Powder*
1	cup dairy-free carob chips
1	cup peanuts

Preheat oven to 350°. Beat egg whites until stiff, gradually adding rice syrup powder. Fold in nuts and carob chips. Drop by teaspoonsful onto paper-covered cookie sheet. Place in oven, turning off heat immediately. Leave in overnight. In the morning, remove from oven, peel off paper. Freezes well. YIELD: 3–4 DOZEN.

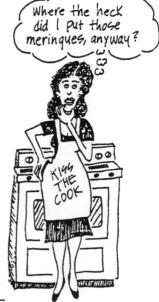

❤ LEMON TWISTS

1	cup	barley flour
1/2	cup	pecans, chopped fine
2/3	cup	*Ohsawa Brown Rice Syrup Powder*
1/2	cup	organic butter, softened
1		egg yolk
11/2	teaspoons	grated lemon peel

Mix flour with pecans and set aside. Beat brown rice syrup powder with butter until fluffy. Beat egg yolk and lemon peel into mixture. Blend mixtures together. Chill in covered bowl for one hour until firm. Flour hands and pull off pieces of dough and roll between palms into 3" strips, then twist like ropes. Place on ungreased cookie sheets abut 1" apart. Bake in preheated 325° oven for about 15 minutes until firm. YIELD: 2 DOZEN COOKIES.

♥ BANANA BREAD

3	ripe bananas, mashed
2	egg whites
1/3	cup high-oleic safflower oil
1/2	cup brown rice syrup
1 1/4	cups Kamut* flour
1	teaspoon baking soda
1	teaspoon non-aluminum baking powder

To mashed bananas, add egg whites, oil, and brown rice syrup. Mix flour with baking soda, baking powder and add to banana mixture. Bake in greased loaf pan in preheated 325° oven for 1 hour. YIELD: 1 LOAF.

*Kamut flour is a type of wheat that many wheat-sensitive persons can tolerate.

♥ TROPICAL FRUITCAKE

2	eggs + 3 egg whites, beaten
1/2	cup high-oleic safflower oil
3/4	cup unsweetened pineapple juice or apple juice concentrate, thawed
	grated orange rind from one large orange
2	cups Kamut* flour
1	cup raw pine nuts
1	cup chopped pecans
1	cup chopped dried prunes
1/2	cup chopped dried papaya
1/2	cup chopped dried apples
1/2	cup raisins

Mix first 5 ingredients together until smooth. Add the remaining ingredients and mix well. Turn into a greased 9" × 5" loaf pan. Bake in a preheated 300° oven for approximately 1 hour. YIELD: 1 LOAF.

Note: To prevent crumbling when slicing, chill first, then use electric knife or very sharp serrated knife.

*Kamut flour is a type of wheat that many wheat-sensitive persons can tolerate.

♥ NO-FAIL PIE CRUST

For one crust:

1   cup whole wheat pastry flour
1/4   teaspoon salt
1/4   cup high-oleic safflower oil
1/8   cup water

Mix flour with salt. Add oil to water, then mix all together. Form into a ball. Place dough between two pieces of waxed paper and roll about 1/8" thick. Put in 8" or 9" pie plate. If heavy fluting is desired, use 8" pie plate. To bake: prick pastry to prevent puffing, place in preheated 475° oven for ten minutes, cool and fill. Double the recipe to make double crust.

♥ APPLE PIE AU NATURÈL

1   double pie crust (see no-fail pie crust above)

FILLING:

1   25 ounce jar unsweetened applesauce
2¹/₂ cups sweet apples, peeled and sliced
1   cup dark raisins
³/₄   teaspoon cinnamon, optional

Mix all filling ingredients together thoroughly. Turn into bottom crust. Cover with top crust pinching edges to seal. Make two or three slits in top to allow steam to escape. Bake in preheated 425° oven for 45–50 minutes. Hint: Make your own applesauce using sweet apples if you are unable to find a sweet tasting, unsweetened applesauce.

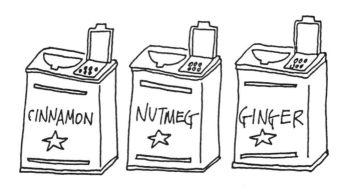

♥ MY FAVORITE UNPUMPKIN PIE

2 1/2 cups sliced carrots, steamed and drained

1/2 cup date sugar or *Ohsawa Brown Rice Syrup Powder*

2 eggs

1/2 teaspoon salt

1/4 teaspoon each cinnamon, nutmeg and ginger

1 3/4 cups *Rice Dream Original Lite Rice Milk*

1/4 cup arrowroot starch

1 unbaked 9" pie shell

Put all filling ingredients into a blender and mix until smooth. Pour into pie shell and bake in preheated 450° oven for 10 minutes. Reduce temperature to 300° and bake an additional 50 minutes, or until knife inserted in filling comes out clean. Cool and serve.

❤ WALNUT-CRACKER PIE

1   cup whole wheat matzoh, finely ground
1   cup walnuts, finely chopped
2   teaspoons non-aluminum baking powder
    pinch of sea salt
3   egg whites
1/2 cup brown rice syrup

Combine first four ingredients in a large bowl and set aside. In small bowl, beat egg whites until stiff, gradually adding syrup so that the egg whites keep their shape. Fold egg mixture into other ingredients and place in oiled 9" pie plate. Bake in preheated 350° oven for 40 minutes. Chill before serving.

♥ ZUCCHINI ICE CREAM

1	medium zucchini, peeled and liquefied in blender to produce 1 cup liquid
4	tablespoons brown rice syrup
1	egg, beaten
1	banana
1/2	cup whipping cream
1	teaspoon vanilla extract, optional

Heat zucchini milk with rice syrup. Add beaten egg and cook over low heat, stirring constantly, until thickened (about 8–10 minutes). Separation may occur, but disregard. Pour mixture in blender and add banana and whir until smooth. Leave in blender to cool. Add whipping cream and vanilla, and blend one minute. Pour into small bowl and freeze until soft ice cream consistency. Beat with electric mixer until smooth and serve. YIELD: 1 PINT.

CANDIES

❤ CAROB PECAN BARK

1   recipe for carob buttercream frosting (see page 63)

1   cup pecan halves or pieces

Thoroughly mix pecans with frosting. Place a piece of wax paper on a cookie sheet and spread mixture with a spatula evenly across to about 1/4" thickness. Place another piece of wax paper over the top of the mixture and smooth the nuts in place by running your hand over it gently, but firmly. Peel off the top piece of paper and place the cookie sheet in the freezer for about an hour. Bark will be firm. Take it out and slice the bark in squares and place in a cellophane bag or other air-tight container. Keep in freezer until serving time, as softening occurs within five minutes after removal from freezer.

Variation: Thoroughly mix chopped or ground nuts with frosting. Fill paper petit-four cups with mixture and freeze same as above. This candy will remain firmer for a longer period of time.

1 CUP WILL YIELD ABOUT 14 CANDIES.

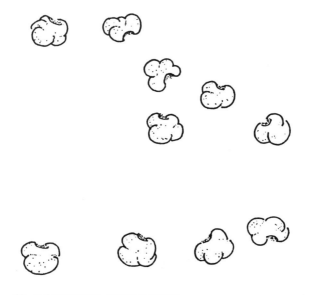

♥ CANDIED POPCORN

1/2   cup melted organic butter
1/2   cup brown rice syrup
3   quarts popped corn
1   cup peanuts

Blend and heat rice syrup and butter. Add nuts, pour over corn and mix well. Spread on cookie sheet. Bake in preheated 350° oven 10–15 minutes until crisp. Rearrange several times while baking to keep from sticking.

WHEAT, SUGAR, DAIRY, AND EGG-FREE DESSERTS

All dessert recipes in this section are wheat-free, sugar-free, dairy-free, and egg-free. Some are also gluten-free as indicated.

❤ **GUILT-FREE CRACKER JACKS**

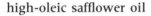

	high-oleic safflower oil
7	cups of 100% organic brown rice cakes, broken into bite-size pieces
1/2	cup 100% organic brown rice syrup, room temperature
3/4	cup organic raw peanuts

Lightly grease a large deep bowl, a sheet cake pan, and a rubber spatula. Place rice cake pieces in bowl. Drizzle syrup over pieces, while stirring with spatula to evenly coat all pieces. Add peanuts and stir to mix well. Pour mixture into pan and spread out using spatula. Bake in preheated 325° oven for 15 minutes until lightly browned. Remove from oven and cool for 5 minutes before removing from pan. Store in a container with a tight-fitting lid. You may have to rinse your hands several times during preparation, but it is well worth it. YIELD: APPROXIMATELY 8 CUPS.

♥ WHEAT-FREE GRANOLA (DESSERT TOPPING)

4	cups rolled oats
1/2	cup sesame seeds
1	cup chopped almonds
1/3	cup apple juice concentrate, thawed
3	tablespoons high-oleic safflower oil
1/3	cup chopped dates or raisins

Mix dry ingredients together, except for fruit. Set aside. Mix wet ingredients together and combine with dry mixture. Mix well. Bake on unoiled sheet pans in preheated 350° oven for 20–25 minutes, stirring occasionally, until browned. Remove from oven and mix in dates or raisins. Let cool, then store in airtight container. Great as a topping for fruit compotes, frozen desserts, and fruit pies, or as a cereal. MAKES APPROXIMATELY 1 1/2 QUARTS.

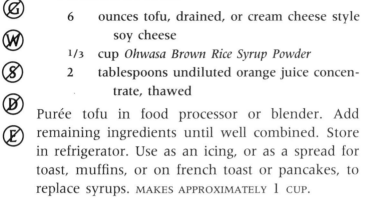

♥ ORANGE BUTTER

6 ounces tofu, drained, or cream cheese style soy cheese

1/3 cup *Ohwasa Brown Rice Syrup Powder*

2 tablespoons undiluted orange juice concentrate, thawed

Purée tofu in food processor or blender. Add remaining ingredients until well combined. Store in refrigerator. Use as an icing, or as a spread for toast, muffins, or on french toast or pancakes, to replace syrups. MAKES APPROXIMATELY 1 CUP.

♥ CRANBERRY-STRAWBERRY JELLO

2 cups frozen strawberries

2 9 ounce jars unsweetened whole cranberry sauce

5 ounces unsweetened strawberry preserves

3 tablespoons agar-agar

Heat first 3 ingredients on medium until berries are thawed. Mix with 3 tablespoons of agar-agar that has been softened in 1/2 cup of water. Boil mixture until agar-agar is dissolved. Pour in 4 cup mold and chill in refrigerator until set. Unmold and serve. SERVES 6.

♥ JELLO CREAM SUPREME

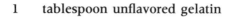
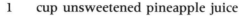

1	tablespoon unflavored gelatin
1	cup unsweetened pineapple juice
3/4	cup fruit-flavored soy yogurt
1/2	cup cold water
1	large or 2 small bananas, mashed well
1	orange, peeled and sectioned, optional

In small sauce pan, sprinkle gelatin over water. Let sit for 5 minutes. Then heat until gelatin is dissolved. Remove from heat and add juice. When cooled, place in blender with the remainder of the ingredients, except orange, and mix until smooth. Pour into mold and refrigerate. Mix in orange sections just before jello sets. SERVES 4.

Note: Yogurt will curdle if liquid is too hot when combined.

❤ CHOCOLATE TAPIOCA PUDDING

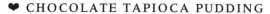

1/2	cup granulated tapioca
21/2	cups *Rice Dream Original Lite Rice Milk*
6	tablespoons *Fruitsource Granulated Sweetener*
1/4	teaspoon sea salt
2/3	cup dairy free chocolate chips (may contain corn and barley)

Combine first four ingredients in a saucepan. Cook on medium heat, stirring continuously just until mixture boils and begins to thicken. Reduce heat and simmer three more minutes while continuing to stir. Remove from heat and quickly mix in chocolate chips until melted. Cool for 5 minutes, then pour into custard cups and chill. SERVES 4.

❤ BANANA-KIWI PUDDING

| 4 | kiwi |
| 5 | medium sized bananas |

I prefer using fruit that has been refrigerated for at least 2 hours. Remove fruit from refrigerator and peel. Cut fruit into chunks and place in food processor or blender. Process until fruit is very smooth and light. Divide pudding into 4 glass dessert cups and serve immediately. SERVES 4.

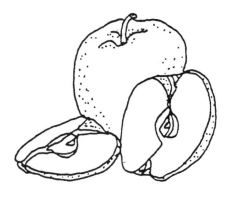

♥ RYE APPLE RAISIN PUDDING

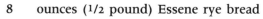
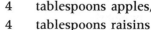

8	ounces (1/2 pound) Essene rye bread
6 1/2	teaspoons *Fruitsource Granular Sweetener*
1/2	teaspoon cinnamon
1/2	teaspoon vanilla
2/3	cup *Rice Dream Original Lite Rice Milk*
4	tablespoons apples, peeled and chopped
4	tablespoons raisins
4	tablespoons chopped walnuts

Break Essene bread into small chunks and place in bowl. Mix dry ingredients and sprinkle on top. Combine vanilla with plain, vanilla, or almond flavored rice milk and pour over bread. Add raisins, apples and walnuts. Mix until well-blended. Divide evenly into 4 custard cups and chill. Serve with a dollop of soy yogurt if desired. SERVES 4.

❤ AMBROSIA

Any amounts of the following:

>   seedless green grapes
>   sliced bananas
>   fresh pineapple chunks
>   shredded coconut, unsweetened
>   apples, sliced, but not peeled
>   mandarin or navel orange sections

Toss in a large bowl with 1/2 pint vanilla soy yogurt, and cool in refrigerator until serving time. Prepare several hours in advance as the fruit juices will sweeten the yogurt. If you have a sweet tooth, add brown rice syrup to yogurt before tossing.

❤ PEACH TAPIOCA PUDDING

1   16 ounce can peaches, packed in water
3   tablespoons fruit juice sweetened peach preserves
1/4 cup granulated tapioca
1/2 teaspoon vanilla
1   cup unsweetened white grape juice

Empty contents of canned peaches into food processor or blender. Add preserves and purée. Remove to a saucepan. Sprinkle peach mixture with tapioca and let sit 5 minutes to soften. Add remaining ingredients, stir to combine. Bring mixture to a quick boil. Reduce heat immediately and cook on medium-low, stirring continuously, until tapioca becomes translucent and mixture thickens. Remove from heat. Cool for 5 minutes before spooning mixture into individual dessert dishes. Refrigerate. SERVES 5.

♥ FRUIT JUICE TAPIOCA

    1/4   cup granulated tapioca
    2   cups unsweetened fruit juice
         brown rice syrup, to taste, optional

Place ingredients together in saucepan and let stand for 5 minutes. Bring to a boil, stirring continuously. Reduce heat immediately, and cook on medium heat, still stirring, until tapioca is translucent and mixture is thickened. Pour into individual dessert dishes and cool in refrigerator.
MAKES 4 SERVINGS.

♥ BANANA-PEACH TAPIOCA PIE

    2   bananas, sliced
    1   recipe Peach Tapioca Pudding (see page 182)
    1   baked pie crust (see pages 82–83 for non-wheat recipes)
    1/2 teaspoon cinnamon
    1   tablespoon *Ohsawa Brown Rice Syrup Powder*

Fold bananas into slightly cooled tapioca pudding and spoon into pie crust. Combine cinnamon and rice syrup powder and sprinkle evenly over the pie. Refrigerate at least 2 hours. YIELD: 1 PIE.

♥ LEMON DREAM CUSTARD OR PIE

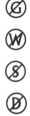

2   cups sugar-free lemonade prepared from *Knudsen* lemonade concentrate

2   packets Knox unflavored gelatin or agar-agar

1   pint *Rice Dream* lemon non-dairy frozen dessert, softened

Pour 1 cup of prepared lemonade into a large saucepan, sprinkle gelatin on top and let stand for 5 minutes. Turn heat to medium-high and stir till gelatin dissolves. Remove liquid from heat and add 1 more cup lemonade and softened frozen dessert till frozen dessert is almost melted. Beat with electric mixer for 1 minute. Chill in individual dessert dishes for custard. (There will be some leftover lemonade. Drink and enjoy!)

For pie, chill until quite thick (about 1 hour). Then spoon into prepared pie shell, placing remaining custard in dessert dishes. Refrigerate until serving time. SERVES 6.

Optional Topping: Lemon zest and unsweetened coconut sprinkled on top before custard completely sets.

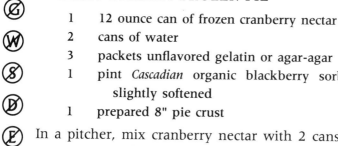

♥ BERRY DELIGHT FROZEN PIE

1	12 ounce can of frozen cranberry nectar
2	cans of water
3	packets unflavored gelatin or agar-agar
1	pint *Cascadian* organic blackberry sorbet, slightly softened
1	prepared 8" pie crust

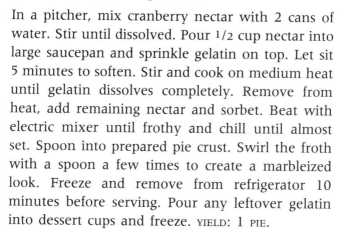

In a pitcher, mix cranberry nectar with 2 cans of water. Stir until dissolved. Pour 1/2 cup nectar into large saucepan and sprinkle gelatin on top. Let sit 5 minutes to soften. Stir and cook on medium heat until gelatin dissolves completely. Remove from heat, add remaining nectar and sorbet. Beat with electric mixer until frothy and chill until almost set. Spoon into prepared pie crust. Swirl the froth with a spoon a few times to create a marbleized look. Freeze and remove from refrigerator 10 minutes before serving. Pour any leftover gelatin into dessert cups and freeze. YIELD: 1 PIE.

♥ APPLE UPSIDE DOWN PIE

(W)
(S)
(D)
(E)

Fill a 7" pie plate with a mixture of:

2	apples, pared and thinly sliced
1/4	cup vanilla soy yogurt
3	heaping teaspoons *Fruitsource Granular Sweetener*
1	teaspoon oat flour

Sprinkle on top, a mixture of:

1/2	cup oat flour
1 1/2	tablespoons high-oleic safflower oil
3	tablespoons *Fruitsource Granular Sweetener*

Place in preheated 350° oven 1/2 or 3/4 hour. Scoop out and serve in dessert bowls. SERVES 4–6.

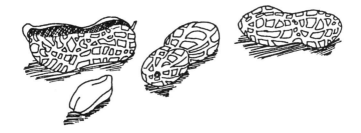

♥ TOFU PEANUT BUTTER PIE

Note: Those with gluten intolerance can use the teff flour pie crust (page 81).

1   *The Simple Soyman* barley pie crust
16   ounces firm tofu
2/3 cup creamy peanut butter
1/4 cup brown rice syrup at room temperature

Bake pie crust according to directions on package. Cool and set aside. Drain and press tofu (see instructions, page 44). Place in blender on high until smooth. Add peanut butter and brown rice syrup. Blend until thoroughly mixed. Fold mixture into baked pie crust. Refrigerate 2 hours before serving.

♥ EASY PEANUT BUTTER GRANOLA BALLS

1/2	cup wheat-free granola (see page 176)
1/2	cup peanut butter
1/2	cup non-fat powdered soy beverage
1/2	cup brown rice syrup or *Fruitsource Liquid Sweetener*

Combine all ingredients and mix thoroughly. Roll into balls (1 1/2" diameter). Refrigerate until firm.
MAKES APPROXIMATELY 36 BALLS.

♥ I-BET-YOU-CAN'T-EAT-JUST-ONE BARLEY BROWNIES

1	cup barley flour
1/2	cup high-oleic safflower oil
1 1/2	bananas, mashed
1/2	cup + 2 tablespoons carob powder
3/4	cup brown rice syrup
1/2	cup carbonated spring water
1/2	cup chopped walnuts
1/4	cup rye flour
1/4	teaspoon salt, optional

Combine dry ingredients and set aside. Beat liquid ingredients together for 1 minute with electric mixer. Then, using a spatula, blend both mixtures together until well blended. Pour batter into a greased 8" square pan and bake in a preheated

350° oven for 30 minutes. Cool and cut into squares. YIELD: 16 SQUARES.

❤ CAROB 3-WAY QUICKIES

    1/2   cup carob powder

    1/2   cup plus 2 tablespoons *Ohsawa Brown Rice Syrup Powder*

    6   ounces vanilla *Rice Dream Original Lite Rice Milk*

    1   teaspoon vanilla

Combine dry ingredients. Gradually stir in milk, blending well. Transfer mixture to a saucepan and bring to boil over medium heat, stirring continuously. Remove from heat and serve as follows:

1. Drizzle over non-dairy frozen dessert as a chocolate sauce alternative, or
2. Mix with vanilla non-dairy beverage to make a chocolate milk alternative, or
3. Mix with thick nut milk (see page 76), heat till thickened, and serve as a chocolate pudding alternative.

MAKES APPROXIMATELY 1 3/4 CUPS.

♥ MELON SORBET

5   cups cubed melons (any combination honey-dew, cantaloupe, or cranshaw)

1/4 cup *Ohsawa Brown Rice Syrup Powder*

2   tablespoons lemon juice

Purée melon cubes in blender. Add syrup powder and lemon juice. Mix well. Spoon mixture into a 13 × 9 × 2 baking dish, cover and freeze, stirring occasionally. Let stand 10–15 minutes before serving. Garnish each serving with a mint leaf.
SERVES 6.

♥ ORANGE AND GRAPEFRUIT SECTIONS

3   grapefruits, peeled and sectioned

3   oranges, peeled and sectioned

1/4 cup fresh orange juice

Ohsawa Brown Rice Syrup Powder, to taste

Place fruit and juice in a bowl and sprinkle rice syrup powder over all. Let set for 1/2 hour, stirring several times. Store in covered jar in refrigerator until serving time. SERVES 8.

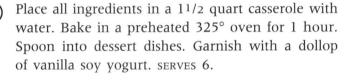

❤ STONED FRUIT COMPOTE

6	ounces dried prunes
6	ounces dried apricots
3/4	cup raisins
21/2	cups water
1/4	cup *Fruitsource Liquid Sweetener*
1	small lemon, sliced thin

Place all ingredients in a 11/2 quart casserole with water. Bake in a preheated 325° oven for 1 hour. Spoon into dessert dishes. Garnish with a dollop of vanilla soy yogurt. SERVES 6.

❤ MOCK GRANOLA TRIFLE

1	cup blackberries
1	cup raspberries
1	cup sliced, canned peaches, well drained
1	cup vanilla soy yogurt
1	cup wheat-free granola (see page 176)

Mix fruit together in a large bowl. Then begin layering in a 11/2 quart glass bowl—first with fruit mixture, then yogurt, ending with granola. Repeat 2 times, reserving 1/3 of the fruit mixture for the top. Looks beautiful served in an attractive glass bowl.

Note: If you have a wheat-free sponge cake on hand, try adding a layer of sponge cake cubes under each fruit layer. SERVES 6.

♥ NON-MILK SHAKE

Base:

Ⓖ Ⓦ Ⓢ Ⓓ Ⓔ

2   scoops vanilla non-dairy frozen dessert
8   ounces low-fat soy or rice non-dairy milk

Place ingredients in blender. Add any one of the following and blend till smooth. SERVES 1.

1   banana
1/2   cup strawberries
1/2   cup raspberries
1/2   cup diced peaches

♥ STRAWBERRY SODA

Ⓖ Ⓦ Ⓢ Ⓓ Ⓔ

2   scoops strawberry non-dairy frozen dessert
6–8   ounces sparkling spring water
3   tablespoons *Knudsen Strawberry Pourable Fruit*

Mix well 1/2 scoop of frozen dessert with 1/2 cup of sparkling water in the bottom of a tall glass. Then add pourable fruit, remaining frozen dessert and sparkling water. Stir gently. SERVES 1.

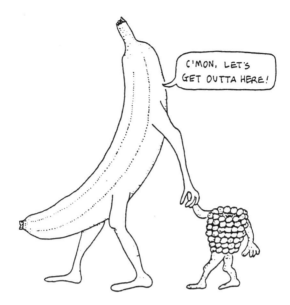

❤ RASPBERRY BANANA SPLIT

1	banana, cut in half lengthwise
2	scoops vanilla Swiss almond non-dairy frozen dessert
1/2	cup raspberries
1/4	cup *Knudsen Pourable Fruit*
1/4	cup wheat-free granola (see page 176)

Place banana slices lengthwise in a banana split dish. Place scoops of frozen dessert on top of bananas. Pour raspberries on top. Spoon pourable fruit over raspberries and top with a sprinkling of granola. Serve in one dish with two spoons. SERVES 2.

♥ MOLDED PEACH SUNDAE

   6   large peaches, peeled and puréed (approximately 1 1/2 cups)

   1   quart vanilla non-dairy frozen dessert

   4   ounces dairy-free chocolate or carob chips

   1   cup toasted almonds

Place all ingredients in a large bowl and stir to mix well. Spoon mixture into a 1 1/2 quart greased mold and freeze until firm. Unmold by quickly dipping the mold in hot water and invert onto a platter. Serve with raspberry pourable fruit. SERVES 6 TO 8.

♥ PEANUT BUTTER ICE MILK

   2 1/2 cups *Rice Dream Original Lite Rice Milk*

   1   cup peanut butter

   3/4   cup brown rice syrup (or more to taste)

Follow ice cream maker's directions, or simply mix all ingredients well in blender and freeze in ice cube trays. Remove from freezer for ten minutes before serving. It will handle like and be as creamy as soda fountain ice cream. YIELD: 1 QUART.

♥ FROZEN PEACH TOFU

1/2	pound tofu
2	sliced peaches
1	teaspoon ginger
1	tablespoon lemon juice
1/4	cup brown rice syrup
1	tablespoon high-oleic safflower oil

Blend all together in food processor until smooth. Freeze until icy, then process again and store in freezer. Blend once again before serving. SERVES 2.

BRAND NAME PRODUCT GUIDE

The following manufacturers may produce more products than those I have listed. However, catalogs are usually available upon request, if they have a mail order business. You may want to request the name of local distributors where their products are sold.

I have included the ingredients listed on the product labels so that you will know in advance if a specific food is acceptable to you. However, **manufacturers continually change ingredients in their products, so always read labels before purchasing.**

❤ BEANS AND PASTAS

American Prairie Organic Beans
Low in salt, wide selection. Lead-free, enamel-lined cans. Distributed by Mercantile Food Company, P.O. Box 1140, Georgetown, CT 06829

Ancient Harvest, 100% Quinoa Pasta, Organic
Corn and wheat free. Quinoa Corporation, P.O. Box 1039, Torrance, CA 90505

Cleopatra's Kamut Pasta
Elbows and thin spaghetti containing organically grown kamut flour and corn flour. Gabriele Macaroni Co., Inc., City of Industry, CA 91748

De Boles Corn Pasta
Corn flour, no preservatives or chemicals added, no salt added. De Boles Nutritional Foods, Inc., Garden City Park, NY 11040

Eden Bi-fun Rice Noodles,
Rice Starch. Eden Foods, Inc., Clinton, MI 49236

Eden Kuzu-Kiri Noodles
Sweet potato starch and kuzu starch. Eden Foods, Inc., Clinton, MI 49236

Eden Soba Noodles
Buckwheat and sea salt. Eden Foods, Inc., Clinton, MI 49236

Foods for Life Rice Elbow Macaroni, Gluten-free.
Brown rice flour, carbohydrate gum. Foods for Life Baking Co., Inc., 3580 Pasadena Ave., Los Angeles, CA 90031

Panda Mung Bean Threads
Mung beans and water. Panda—Eastimpex, San Francisco, CA 94126

Pastariso Rice Pasta, Organic
100% brown rice—elbows, spaghetti, twists.

Pastariso Products, Inc., 55 Ironside Crescent, Units 6 and 7, Scarborough, Ontario, Canada M1X 1N3

Vita-Spelt Pasta, 100% Organic
No eggs or oils—shells, rotini, elbows, spaghetti. Purity Foods, Inc. 2871 West Jolly Rd., Okemos, MI 48864

Walnut Acres, Kidney Beans, Organic
Well water, salt-free (cans). Walnut Acres, Pennscreek, PA 17862

❤ BEVERAGES

Bambú Instant Coffee Substitute
Chicory, figs, wheat, malted barley, acorns; no coffee, chocolate or caffeine. Bioforce of America Ltd., Plainview, NY 11803

Cafe Altura Coffee, Organic
Naturally low in caffeine. Terra Nova Clean Foods, Inc., P.O. Box 1647, Ojai, CA 93023

Cafix Coffee Substitute—Instant caffeine-free
Roasted malt, chicory, barley, rye, beet root, figs. Imported by: Richter Bros. Inc., Carlstadt, NJ 07072

Dacopa—Instant Coffee Substitute
100% roasted dahlia syrup. No caffeine, additives or preservatives. Dacopa Foods, a division of

California Natural Products, P.O. Box 1219, Lathrop, CA 95330

Knudsen Tomato Juice
Pure spring water, pure tomato juice from organic tomato concentrate, organic lemon juice concentrate, sea salt, (glass jar). Knudsen & Sons, Inc., Chico, CA 95928

Roastaroma—Instant Grain Beverage
Roasted barley, crystal malt, roasted chicory root, roasted carob, cassia bark, allspice and star anise. No artificial colorings, flavorings or preservatives. Celestial Seasonings, Inc., 4600 Sleepytime Dr., Boulder, CO 80301-3292

Yannoh, Instant Grain Beverage
Organically grown barley, rye, malted barley, chicory, and non-organic acorns. Distributed by Eden Foods, Inc., Clinton, MI 49236

♥ BREADSTUFFS

Arrowhead Mills Teff Flour, Organic Whole Grain
Arrowhead Mills, Inc., Box 2059, Hereford, TX 79045

Dimpflmeier Rye Bread, Unyeasted
Rye flour, spring water, sourdough starter, salt.

Dimpflmeier Bakery Ltd., 32 Advance Road, Toronto, Ontario, Canada M8Z 2T4

Edward & Sons Brown Rice Snaps, Gluten-free
Brown rice and sesame seeds. Edward & Sons, Carpinteria, CA 93013

Floridor Rye Crisp Crackers, Unyeasted
Whole grain rye flour and spring water, no preservatives, coloring or artificial ingredients. Distributor: Lifetone International, One South Ocean Blvd., Boca Raton, FL 33432

Garden of Eatin' Tortillas
Unyeasted whole wheat flour, water, aluminum-free baking powder, soybean oil, and sea salt. Garden of Eatin', Inc., Los Angeles, CA 90029

Health Valley Rice Bran Crackers, Gluten-free
Brown rice, corn, soy, apple-pineapple juice, soy flour and soy oil, pear-pineapple juice, honey, rice bran oil and rice bran, almond and vanilla, soy lecithin, baking soda, lemon juice. Health Valley Foods, Inc., 16100 Foothill Blvd., Irwindale, CA 91706-7811

Holgrain Brown Rice Crackers, Gluten-free
Natural brown rice only. Parco Foods, Inc., Blue Island, IL 60406

Jaclyn's Breadcrumbs
Organic whole wheat flour, water, yeast, safflower

oil, sea salt, barley malt. Jacklyn's Food Products, Inc., P.O. Box 1314, Cherry Hill, NJ 08034

Ka·me Rice Crackers
Rice, corn oil. Unsalted. Shaffer Clarke & Co., Inc., Darien, CT 06820

Kavli Norwegian Flatbread (Crackers)
Whole rye, yeast, salt. O. Kavli A/S, P.O. Box 435, N. 5001 Bergen, Norway

Lundberg Rice Cakes
Organically-grown whole-grain brown rice, unsalted; no artificial colors, flavors, or preservatives. Lundberg Family Farms, P. O. Box 369, Richvale, CA 95974-0369

Pritikin English Muffins
Whole wheat flour, water, cornmeal, wheat grits, yeast, raisin juice concentrate, 2% or less salt, lactic acid, acetic acid, ascorbic acid; no artificial preservatives, colors, or flavors. Interstate Brands Corp., Kansas City, MO 64111

Pritikin Whole Wheat Bread
100% stone ground whole wheat flour, water, unsweetened raisin juice, yeast, salt, bran. Interstate Brands Corp., Kansas City, MO 64111

Wasa Rye Crackers, Gluten-free
Whole grain rye, salt, yeast. Liberty Richter, Saddle Brook, NJ 07662

Bickford Vanilla

Concentrated vanilla, contains no alcohol, sugar, salt. Bickford Laboratories Co., 282 S. Main St., Akron, OH 44308

Cook's Vanilla Powder

Vanilla bean extractives in a dextrose (sugar) base. No preservatives or artificial ingredients. No alcohol. Almond powder is available also. Cook Flavoring Co., P.O. Box 890, Tacoma, WA 98401

Corning Cookware

"Visions" line without non-stick coating. Call 1-800-999-3436

Eden Kuzu Root Starch

100% kuzu, no added potato starch. Eden Foods, Inc., Clinton, MI 49236

Ener-G Foods Egg Replacer

Potato starch, tapioca flour, methylcellulose, calcium carbonate, citric acid. Ener-G Foods Inc., P.O. Box 84887, Seattle, WA 98124-5787

If You Care Baking Cups, 100% Unbleached (dioxin-free)

Imported by: A. V. Olsson Trading Co., Inc., Greenwich, CT 06831

If You Care Baking Paper, 100% Unbleached
Imported by: Laharco Holdings, Ltd., 180 Bloor St.
  West, Toronto, Ontario, Canada M5S 2V6

Melitta Coffee Filters, 100% Unbleached
Melitta, Cherry Hill, NJ 08003, 1-800-451-1694

Menominee Paper, Waxed, Natural
No dioxin producing chlorine or bleaching agents
  used in processing. Good for microwave use.
  Menominee Paper Co., Subsidiary of Bell Fibre
  Products, Menominee, MI 49858

Muir Glen Tomato Products, Organic
Purées, sauces, chunks, pastes. No chemical additives or preservatives. Lead-free enamel lined
  cans. Muir Glen, P.O. Box 1498, Sacramento,
  CA 95812

Natural Brew Coffee Filters, 100% Unbleached
Natural Brew, Rockline, Inc., P.O. Box 1007, She-
  boygan, WI 53082-1007

Niblack Carob Powder
No preservatives or additives. Niblack Foods, Inc.,
  Rochester, NY 14608

Seventh Generation Paper Products, 100% Unbleached
Including paper towels, napkins. Seventh Generation, Colchester, VT 05446-1672. 1-800-456-
  1177 for catalog

Sunspire Carob and Chocolate Chips, Dairy and Sugar-free

Many varieties to choose from. Read label for precise ingredients. Sunspire, San Leandro, CA 94577

♥ COOKING OILS AND CONDIMENTS

Bragg Liquid Aminos

Essential amino acids from soybeans only. Live Food Products, Inc., Box 7, Santa Barbara, CA 93102

Dr. Bronner's Bouillon, Mineral

Soya bouillon base, blackstrap molasses, vitamin C, lemon and orange juice solids, soya lecithin (oil-free), ocean dulse, papain enzymes (glass jar). Rabbi Emanuel H. Bronner, Assoc., SMMC, DD, Box 28, Escondido, CA 92025

Eden Soy Sauce—"Tamari"

Water, soybeans, sea salt, alcohol (not listed on label). Eden Foods, Inc., Clinton, MI 49236

Frontier Herbs, 100% Organic Spices, Non-Irradiated

A wide variety (glass jars). Frontier Herbs, Norway, IA 52318

John Wood's Sauerkraut

Organic fresh cabbage, pure salt, water (glass jar).

John Wood Farms, John Wood Products, Suamico, WI 54173

L'Estornell Olive Oil, Organic Extra-Virgin
(glass bottle) Imported by: VEA N. A. Inc., Waukeegan, IL 60085

Real Salt
Mined from rock sea salt deposit in Redmond Utah. No anti-caking agents. American Orsa, Inc., Redmond, Utah 84652

Spectrum Apple Cider Vinegar, Organic
Raw, unpasteurized (glass jar). Spectrum Naturals, Inc., 133 Copeland St., Petaluma, CA 94952

Spectrum Oils, Organic Cooking
An assortment of organic, cold-pressed, unrefined cooking oils, including extra-virgin olive oil and high-oleic safflower oil (glass bottles). Spectrum Marketing, Inc., Petaluma, CA 94952

Walnut Acres No-Yolk Mayonnaise
Canola oil, pasteurized egg whites (with guar gum), organic apple cider, alfalfa honey, salt, pepper, mustard (glass jar). Walnut Acres, Pennscreek, PA 17862

Alta-Dena Kefir

Cultured pasteurized Grade A milk, nonfat milk, cream, lactobacillus caucasicus, lactobacillus acidophilus, lactobacillus bulgaricus culture. Alta-Dena Dairy, City of Industry, CA 91744

Alta-Dena Kefir Cheese

Pasteurized Grade A Milk, cream, lactobacillus caucasicus and salt. Alta-Dena Dairy, City of Industry, CA 91744

Coach Farms Yogurt, Goat's Milk

No additives of any kind. Coach Farms, Inc., Pine Plains, NY 12567

Coach Farms Yogurt Drink, Goat's Milk

Yo-Goat cultured goat's milk drink. Pasteurized grade A goat's milk. No additives of any kind. Coach Farms, Inc., Pine Plains, NY 12567

Hollow Road Farms Yogurt, Sheep's Milk, Organic

Handmade of pasteurized sheep's milk and active yogurt culture. No preservatives, sugar, salt, stabilizers, or other additives. Hollow Road Farms, Stuyvesant, NY 12173

Horizon Yogurt, Organic

Fat-free yogurt, organic pasteurized skim milk, skim milk powder, natural flavor, pectin, active

yogurt cultures. Natural Horizons, Boulder, CO
80301

Nutquick Almond Milk Powder
99% blanched almond meal, 1% guar gum.
Ener-G Foods, Inc., P.O. Box 84887, Seattle, WA
98124-5787

Pacific Foods Soy Beverage
Water, organic soybeans, no malt sweeteners (5
grams of fat per 8 ounce serving). Ideal for gluten intolerants (aseptic packaging). Pacific Foods
of Oregon, Inc., Tvalatin, OR 97062

Purity Farms Ghee, Organic
Clarified butter. No preservatives, coloring or salt
(glass jars). Regular style organic butter also.
Purity Farms, Inc., Lancaster, MA 01523

Rice Dream Original Lite Rice Milk
1% fat, non-dairy beverage. Filtered water, organic
brown rice, expeller-pressed high-oleic safflower oil,
sea salt, 2 grams fat per 8 ounce serving. Imagine
Foods, Inc., 299 California Ave., Palo Alto, CA 94306

Walnut Acres Milk, Skim, Powdered, Organic
Only source of organic powdered skim milk available. Walnut Acres, Pennscreek, PA 17862

White Wave Yogurt, Dairyless
Plain or fruited, organically grown soybeans,

brown rice syrup, unmodified tapioca starch, pectin, guar gum, carrageenan, citric acid. White Wave, Inc., Boulder, CO 80303

♥ DESSERTS

Ben & Jerry's Ice Cream
Skim milk, cream, sugar, egg yolks, vanilla extract, partially hydrogenated soybean oil, guar gum, carrageenan, salt, baking soda, soy lecithin. P.O. Box 240, Waterbury, VT 05676

Breyers Ice Cream
Milk, cream, sugar, butter, salt, natural flavors. Kraft, Inc., Philadelphia, PA 19104

Cascadian Farms Fruit Sorbet, Organic, Dairy-free
Fruit sweetened. Contains fruit, grape juice concentrate, water, fruit pectin. Cascadian Farms, Rockport, WA 98283

Dream Pudding Carob, Non-dairy, Fat-free
Water, brown rice syrup, rice starch, carob, carrageenan, vanilla, sea salt. Imagine Foods, Inc., 350 Cambridge Ave., Palo Alto, CA 94306

Häagen-Dazs Ice Cream
No artificial flavor, colorings, stabilizers, emulsifiers, additives, preservatives, or added salt. Fresh

cream, skim milk, sugar, egg yolk, natural
vanilla. Häägen-Dazs Co., Teaneck, NJ 07666

Ice Bean Frozen Dessert
No refined sweeteners. Water, soybeans, honey,
soy oil, soy lecithin, carob bean and guar, flavorings (assorted flavors—contents may vary).
Farm Foods, Summertown, TN 38483

Rice Dream Frozen Dessert
Well water, rice, sesame tahini, maple syrup, Irish
moss, guar gum, flavorings. Imagine Foods, Inc.,
299 California Ave., Palo Alto, CA 94306

The Simple Soyman Pie Crust, Frozen
Dairy and wheat free. Organic barley flour, organic
brown rice flour, water, tofu, soy oil, sea salt.
The Simple Soyman, Milwaukee, WI 53209-
0771

❤ FRUITS AND PRESERVES

Cascadian Farms Fruits, Assorted Frozen
Organic fruit only. Cascadian Farms, Rockport,
WA 98283

Eden Apple Butter
Apples and apple cider. Eden Foods, Inc., Clinton,
MI 49236

Eden Applesauce

Apples and water. No additives. Eden Foods, Inc., Clinton, MI 49236

Knudsen Organic Fruit Spreads

Grape juice concentrate, fruit, pectin, lemon juice concentrate. No preservatives, artificial colors or flavoring. Knudsen & Sons, Inc. Chico, CA 95928

Sonoma Cranberries, Dried

Dried cranberries, sucrose (sugar), cranberries, cranberry juice from concentrate. No sulfur. Timber Crest Farms, 4791 Dry Creek Rd., Healdburg, CA 95448

Sorrell Ridge Spreadable Fruit

Assorted flavors, fruit juice sweetened spreadable fruit containing; fruit, unsweetened fruit juices, and pectin (glass jar). Sorrell Ridge Farm, 100 Market Street, Port Reading, NJ 07064

❤ MISCELLANEOUS

Poplite Popcorn, Organic Microwave

100% organic yellow popcorn. Country Grown Foods, 12202 Woodbine, Redford, MI 48239

Vermont Country Store Maple Butter

100% pure (glass jar). Vermont Country Store, Weston, VT 05161

Wolff's Kasha—roasted buckwheat
No additives, fortifiers or preservatives. Wolff's—
  Birkett Mills, Penn Yan, NY 14527

❤ NUT BUTTERS

Arrowhead Mills Peanut Butter, certified aflatoxin-free
Deaf Smith peanut butter. 100% Valencia peanuts,
  no pesticides or herbicides. Arrowhead Mills,
  Inc., Box 2059, Hereford, TX 79045

Walnut Acres Peanut Butter, Organic, certified aflatoxin-free
Smooth or crunchy, salted or unsalted available.
  US #1 unblanched peanuts. Walnut Acres, Pennscreek, PA 17862

Westbrae Cashew Nut Butter
Roasted cashews. Westbrae Natural Foods, Berkeley, CA 94706

❤ SWEETENERS

Fruitsource™, Powdered or Liquid
Powdered—metal cylinder, liquid—glass jar. Unrefined grape juice concentrate and whole rice
  syrup, Fruitsource, 1803 Mission St., Ste. 404,
  Santa Cruz, CA 95060

Knudsen Pourable Fruit
In 5 flavors. No refined sugar. Knudsen & Sons, Inc., Chico, CA 95928

Ohsawa Brown Rice Syrup Powder
Distributed by: Gold Mine Natural Food Co., San Diego, CA 92102

Shady Maple Farms Maple Syrup
Organically produced and packaged, no formaldehyde added. Shady Maple Farms. La Guadeloupe, Quebec, Canada G0M 1G0

Sucanat Organic 100% Evaporated Sugar Cane Juice
No additives, no preservatives. Pronatec Corporation, P.O. Box 780, 35 Ash St., Hollis, NH 03049

Vermont Country Store Maple Sugar Granules
Powdered maple sugar—guaranteed genuine 100% pure. Vermont Country Store, Weston, VT 05161

INDEX

Mayodelicious, 68
Mayonnaise, 67, 68
MAYONNAISE, WALNUT ACRES
    NO-YOLK DRESSING, 68,
    112, 124, 205
MELITTA COFFEE FILTERS, 6, 203
Melon Sorbet, 190
MENOMINEE WAXED PAPER, 6,
    203
Meringue, 69
Meringue pie crusts, 82
Milk, cow's, 69; also see almond,
    artichoke, buttermilk, choco-
    late, evaporated, goat's, non-
    fat, nut, powdered, sesame
    seed, sour, soy, sweetened con-
    densed, whole
MILK, ENER-G FOODS, POW-
    DERED ALMOND, 207
MILK, PACIFIC FOODS SOY, 207
MILK, RICE DREAM ORIGINAL
    LITE, 71, 113, 118, 133, 134,
    142, 147, 149, 170, 179, 180,
    189, 194, 207
MILK, WALNUT ACRES POW-
    DERED, 207
Millet, 21, 97
Miso, 21, 84
Miso, barley, 34
Miso, red, 35
Miso, white, 34, 35
Mock graham crackers, 37
Mock granola trifle, 191
Mock iced coffee, 49
Mock sour cream, 52
Molasses, 22, 51, 94
Molded peach sundae, 194
Monte Cristo sandwich bake, 142
MUFFINS, PRITIKIN ENGLISH, 201
MUIR GLEN TOMATO PRODUCTS,
    203
Mung bean threads, 22, 78, 197
My Egg-Free Mayo, 163
My Favorite Unpumpkin Pie, 170

NATURAL BREW COFFEE FIL-
    TERS, 203
NIBLACK CAROB POWDER,
    203

No-cook catsup, 161
No-fail pie crust, 168
Non-fat milk, 55
Non-milk shake, 192
Nut burgers supreme, 153
Nut butters, see almond, cashew,
    peanut, pecan, pumpkin seed,
    soybean tahini
Nut loaf/stuffing, 155
Nut milks, 76
Nut pie crust, 82
NUTQUICK ALMOND MILK POW-
    DER, 76, 207

Oat bran, 22, 96
Oat flour, 97
OHSAWA BROWN RICE SYRUP
    POWDER, 53, 76, 93, 121,
    141, 164, 165, 170, 177, 183,
    189, 190, 212
Oils: see canola, corn, olive, peanut,
    sesame, sunflower, BRAND
    NAME PRODUCT GUIDE, 205
Olive oil, 13, 50
Orange and grapefruit sections, 190
Orange butter, 177
Orange juice, 89
Orzo pasta, 97

PACIFIC FOODS SOY BEVERAGE,
    71, 74, 207
Pancake syrup, 78
PAPER PRODUCTS, 6, 202–203
PANDA MUNG BEAN THREADS,
    78, 197
Pasta (white flour), 78; also see:
    brown rice, buckwheat noo-
    dles (soba), corn, mung
    beanthreads, quinoa, rice,
    spelt, sweet potato noodles
    (kuzu-kiri), tofu, BRAND
    NAME PRODUCT GUIDE, 196,
    197, 198
PASTARISO RICE PASTA, 197
Pastry flour, 51, 96
Peach tapioca pudding, 182
Peanut butter, 79, 211
Peanut butter ice milk, 194

-217-